RECI
FOR VEGAN
LOVERS

Original recipes for eating well without meat

Sarah Miller

Table of Contents

TABLESPOON CONVERSIONS

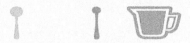

TABLESPOON   TEASPOON   CUP

Tablespoons to one cup, half cup, quarter cup and more.

3 TEASPOONS = 1 TABLESPOON

1 TABLESPOON = 1/16 CUP

2 TABLESPOONS + 2 TEASPOONS = 1/6 CUP

2 TABLESPOONS = 1/8 CUP

4 TABLESPOONS = 1/4 CUP

5 TABLESPOONS + 1 TEASPOON = 1/3 CUP

6 TABLESPOONS = 3/8 CUP

8 TABLESPOONS = 1/2 CUP

10 TABLESPOONS + 2 TEASPOONS = 2/3 CUP

12 TABLESPOONS = 3/4 CUP

16 TABLESPOONS = 1 CUP

tbsp.

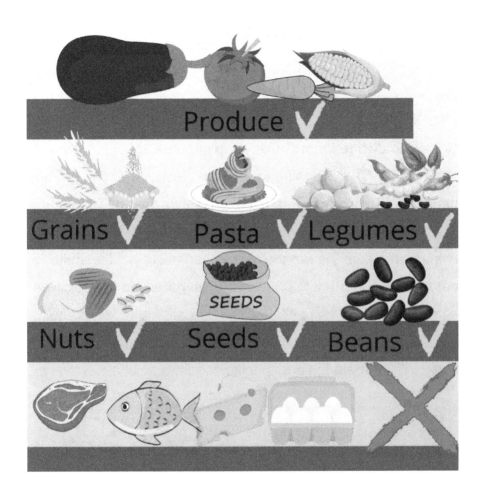

Introduction

So you've decided that you'd like to become vegan, but where do you start? Transitioning to a vegan lifestyle can seem really daunting but often the idea of a big lifestyle change is a lot scarier than actually doing it. If you focus on making one change at a time the progression to veganism will feel quite natural. It's important to go at your own pace and to decide on a method that works best for you. Here are some ideas and guidelines to structure your transition to veganism, just be sure to tailor them to your specific needs.

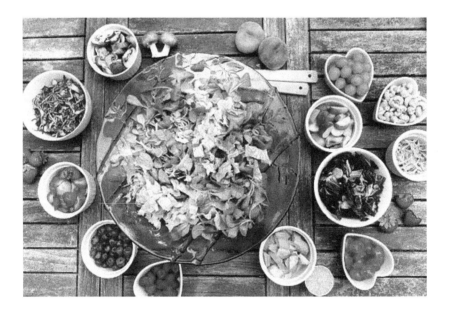

Learn as much as you can

Before you even begin the transition the first step is to start familiarizing yourself with veganism. This will really help you feel prepared and knowledgeable as you begin changing your lifestyle.

- **Learn the benefits of a vegan lifestyle** and educate yourself about the practices and costs behind the production of animal products. Find your own personal reasons for being vegan, there's loads of them.

- **Learn how to optimally nourish your body on a plant-based diet.**

- Start reading ingredients lists - **Learn how to tell if a product is vegan** and familiarize yourself with the less obvious animal derived ingredients that show up in unsuspecting products.

- Be on the lookout for vegan products at your local grocery store, research vegan friendly restaurants and grocery stores in your area.

- Read, watch, learn. Seek out vegan documentaries, books, magazines, websites, blogs, forums, and people. They can offer valuable insights, support, and will help you to feel more confident in your transition.

Add to your diet before you subtract from it

- Begin incorporating more whole grain, beans, legumes, nuts, seeds, and tofu into your diet. Familiarize yourself with their preparation, storage, and uses.

- Start collecting and experimenting with vegan recipes that appeal to you.

- Find a few different quick and easy vegan meals that you enjoy and get comfortable preparing them.

- Switch out milk for a non-dairy alternative such as almond or soy. This is an easy switch for most people but there's a lot of options, so experiment to find which you like best.

There is a huge difference between adopting a vegan lifestyle and "going on a diet". It's easy to be tempted into straying from diet plan or "cheating", but it's not the same with veganism. When you know exactly why you want to be vegan you simply don't stray from the lifestyle. This is why it is so important to learn the benefits of a vegan lifestyle and the effect animal products have on our health, environment, and humanity. Once you've taken the time to open your eyes to the real effects animal products have on our lives it just sticks with you and there's no going back on that.

VEGAN RECIPES TO A VEGAN LIFESTYLE

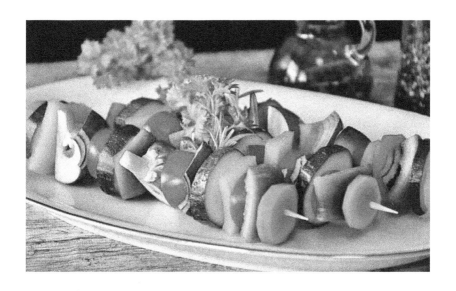

Vegan Refried Beans

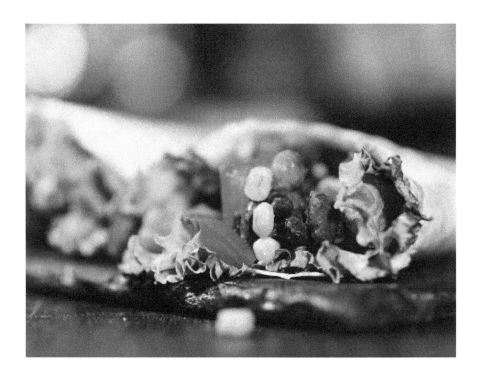

Ingredients

1 tablespoon olive oil1 onion, diced
1 (15 ounce) can pinto beans,drained
3 tablespoons tomato pastechili powder to taste
1 cup vegetable broth

Directions

Heat oil in a medium skillet over medium heat. Saute
onions untiltender. Stir in beans, tomato paste, chili
powder and vegetable broth. Cook 5 minutes, or until
stock has reduced. Mash with a potato masher.

Vegan Carrot Soup

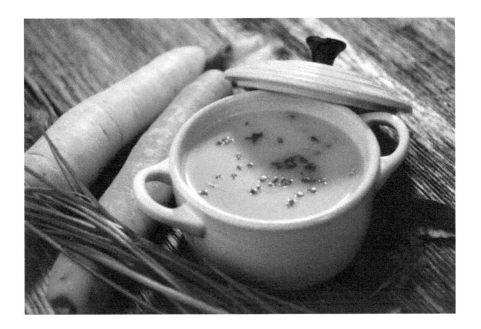

Ingredients

- 1 tablespoon vegetable oil1 large onion, diced
- 3 cloves garlic, minced4 large carrots, sliced
- 5 new potatoes, quartered2 cups vegetable broth
- 2 teaspoons grated fresh ginger1 teaspoon curry powder
- salt and pepper to taste

Directions

- Heat oil in a soup pot over medium heat. Add onion and garlic, and cook stirring often until onion is translucent. Add carrots and potatoes, and cook for just a few minutes to allow the carrots to sweat out some of their juices.

- Pour the vegetable broth into the pot, and season with ginger, currypowder, salt and pepper. Bring to a boil, then reduce heat to low.
- Simmer for 15 to 20 minutes, until carrots are tender.

- Puree soup in small batches using a food processor or blender, or ifyou have an immersion blender, it can be done in the soup pot.
- Reheat soup if necessary, and serve.

Vegan Pancakes

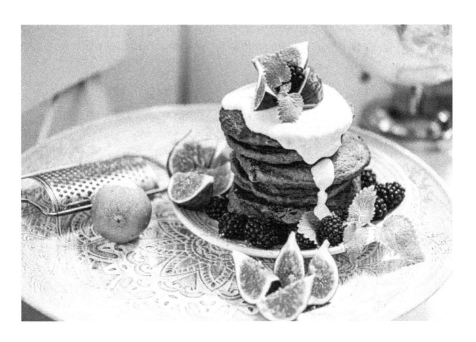

Ingredients

- 1 1/4 cups all-purpose flour
- 2 tablespoons white sugar
- 2 teaspoons baking powder
- 1/2 teaspoon salt
- 1 1/4 cups water
- 1 tablespoon oil

Directions

- Sift the flour, sugar, baking powder, and salt into a large bowl. Whisk the water and oil together in a small bowl. Make a well in thecenter of the dry ingredients, and pour in the wet. Stir just until blended; mixture will be lumpy.

- Heat a lightly oiled griddle over medium-high heat. Drop batter by large spoonfuls onto the griddle, and cook until bubbles form andthe edges are dry. Flip, and cook until browned on the other side.Repeat with remaining batter.

Vegan Casserole

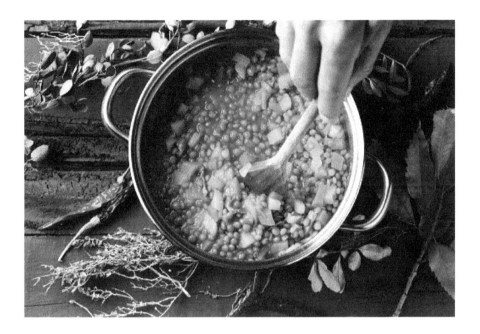

Ingredients

- 5 russet potatoes, peeled
- 1 clove crushed garlic
- 1 stalk celery, chopped
- 1 bunch fresh parsley, chopped8 whole black peppercorns
- 1 onion, chopped
- 1 bay leaf
- 1 tablespoon light miso paste1 tablespoon olive oil

- 1 tablespoon olive oil 3/4 cup diced red onion1 clove garlic, minced
- 1/2 pound fresh mushrooms,sliced
- 1 pound firm tofu, crumbled

- 4 tablespoons hickory flavoredbarbecue sauce
- 1 tablespoon nutritional yeast(optional)
- 1 tablespoon vegetarian chickenflavored gravy mix
- 1 teaspoon paprika
- tablespoon tamari

- cup fresh corn kernels1 cup chopped spinach

- tablespoons olive oil
- 1/8 cup whole wheat pastry flour2 teaspoons nutritional yeast (optional)
- 1 tablespoon vegetarian chickenflavored gravy mix
- 1 cube vegetable bouillon

Directions

- Preheat oven to 400 degrees F (200 degrees C).

- Peel and quarter potatoes. Place in a medium or large size pot withwater to cover. Add garlic, celery, parsley, peppercorns, onion, andbay leaf. Bring to a boil, cover, and simmer over medium-low heat for 15 to 20 minutes or until potatoes are very tender.

- To Make Filling: While potatoes are cooking, in a large skillet heat 1 tablespoon oil and saute onion and garlic. Saute for 1 minute over medium heat, then add mushrooms and saute for 2 minutes.

- Crumble tofu in chunks into the skillet and saute briefly, mixing well. Stir in barbecue sauce, yeast, gravy mix, thyme, paprika, and tamari. Mix well and saute, stirring frequently, for 20 minutes over medium heat.

- Transfer potatoes from water to a large bowl, reserving 3 1/2 cups of the remaining stock. Add miso, oil, and 3/4 to 1 cup of the potato stock to the potatoes a little at a time, mashing potatoes as you add the stock. Add only enough water to moisten potatoes adequately. Do not over moisten, this potato mixture will be the crust covering of the casserole.

- Add corn and spinach to filling mixture and mix well. Spoon filling into an oiled, shallow ovenproof casserole dish. Pat down with back of a large spoon. Spread potato crust evenly over filling, smoothing top with a spoon or spatula. Dust evenly with paprika. Bake for 30 to 40 minutes, or until crust is golden.

- While casserole bakes, prepare gravy. Heat oil in a large frying pan. Add flour and yeast, stir with a whisk over medium heat to form a paste. Slowly stir in 2 1/2 cups of reserved potato water, whisking as you stir to allow gravy to thicken. Stir in instant gravy mix and continue whisking until gravy is thick and smooth; add additional potato water, if necessary. Serve casserole with crust on the bottom and filling on top. Spoon gravy over top.

Harvest Vegan Nut Roast

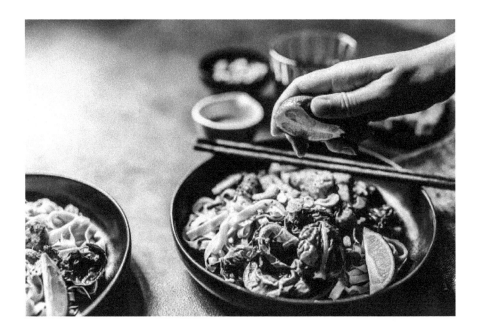

Ingredients

- 1/2 cup chopped celery
- 2 onions, chopped
- 3/4 cup walnuts
- 3/4 cup pecan or sunflower meal
- 2 1/2 cups soy milk
- 1 teaspoon dried basil
- 1 teaspoon dried oregano
- 3 cups bread crumbs
- salt and pepper to taste

Directions

- Preheat oven to 350 degrees F (175 degrees C). Lightly oil a loafpan.

- In a medium size frying pan, saute the chopped celery and theonion in 3 teaspoons water until cooked.

- In a large mixing bowl combine the celery and onion with walnuts,pecan or sunflower meal, soy milk, basil, oregano, bread crumbs,salt and pepper to taste; mix well. Place mixture in the prepared loaf pan.

- Bake for 60 to 90 minutes; until the loaf is cooked through.

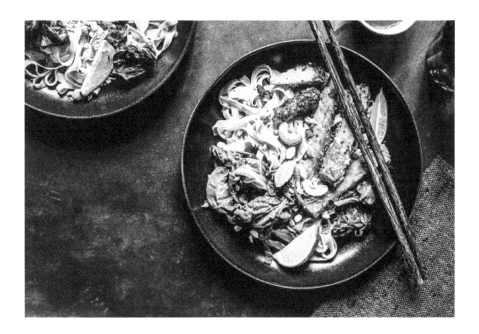

Vegan Davy Crockett Bars

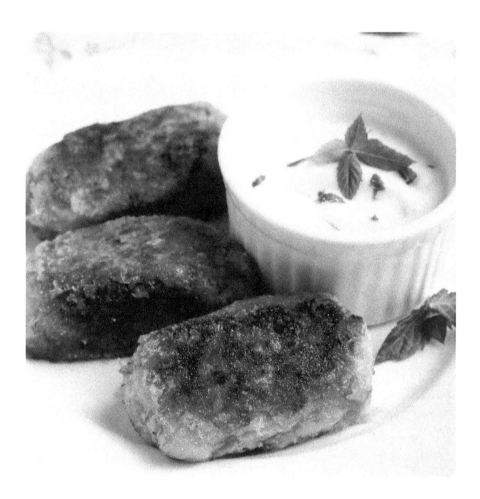

Ingredients

- 2 cups all-purpose flour
- 1 cup white sugar
- 1 teaspoon salt
- teaspoon baking powder1 teaspoon baking soda

- cup brown sugar
- cups quick cooking oats

- 1 cup vegan chocolate chips
- 1 teaspoon vanilla extract
- 3/4 cup vegetable oil

Directions

- Preheat an oven to 350 degrees F (175 degrees C).

- Mix flour, sugar, salt, baking powder, and baking soda together in alarge bowl. Stir in brown sugar, oats, and chocolate chips. In a separate bowl, combine oil and vanilla extract; stir into flour mixture.Press dough into a 15x10 inch jelly roll pan.

- Bake in the preheated oven until lightly brown, about 15 minutes.Cool before cutting into bars.

Creamy Vegan Corn Chowder

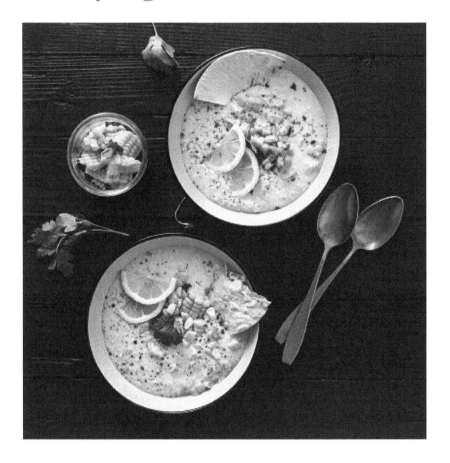

Ingredients

- 2 tablespoons olive oil 1 small onion, chopped
- 1 cup celery, chopped 1 cup carrots, chopped
- 1 clove garlic, minced
- 2 1/2 cups water
- 2 cubes vegetable bouillon
- 2 cups corn
- 2 cups soy milk
- 1 tablespoon flour
- 1 teaspoon dried parsley 1 teaspoon garlic powder

- 1 teaspoon salt
- 1 teaspoon pepper

Directions

Heat oil in a large skillet over medium heat. Stir in onions and celery;cook until just slightly golden. Stir in carrots and garlic; cook until garlic is slightly golden.

Meanwhile, bring water to a boil over high heat. Stir in bouillon, andreduce heat to medium. When bouillon cubes have dissolved, add corn and the vegetables from the skillet. Cook until vegetables are tender. Add water, if necessary. Reduce heat to low, and pour in 1 cup soy milk. Stir soup well, then stir in remaining 1 cup soy milk.
Quickly whisk in flour. Stir in parsley, garlic powder, salt, and pepper. Cook, stirring constantly, until chowder thickens, about 15to 20 minutes.

'Dark Night' Vegan Chocolate Mousse

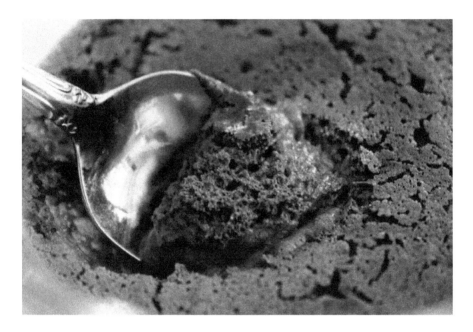

Ingredients

- 1 (16 ounce) package silken tofu, drained
- 3/4 cup Stevia Extract In TheRaw® Cup For Cup

- teaspoon pure vanilla extract
- 1 tablespoon light agave syrup
- 1/4 cup soy milk
- 1/2 cup unsweetened cocoapowder

- tablespoons carob powderMint leaves

Directions

- Place tofu, Stevia Extract In The Raw and vanilla in a food processor or blender. Process until well blended. Add remainingingredients and process until mixture is fully blended.

- Pour into small dessert cups or espresso cups. Chill for at least 2hours. Garnish with fresh mint leaves just before serving.

Vegan Peanut Butter Fudge

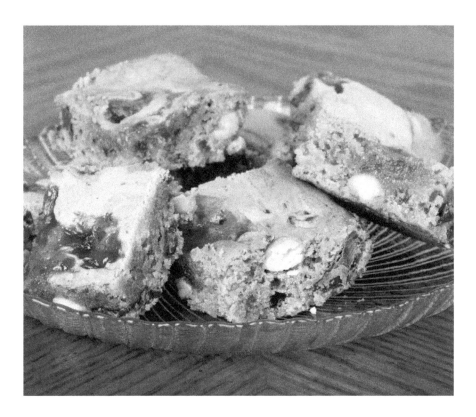

Ingredients

- 2 cups packed brown sugar
- 1/8 teaspoon salt
- 3/4 cup soy milk
- 2 tablespoons light corn syrup
- 4 tablespoons peanut butter
- 1 teaspoon vanilla extract

Directions

- Lightly grease one 9x5x2 inch pan.

- In a 2-quart pot over very low heat, mix together the brown sugar, salt, soy milk, corn syrup, peanut butter and vanilla. Cook until hotand brown sugar is dissolved.

- Quickly pour into pan and refrigerate. Cut into squares and store insemi-airtight container in refrigerator.

Creamy Vegan Hot Cocoa

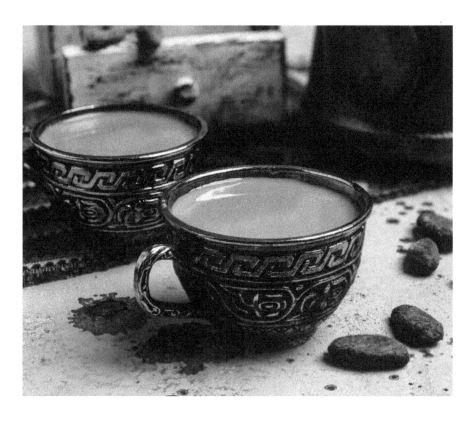

Ingredients

- tablespoons canned coconutmilk
- 1/2 teaspoon vanilla extract
- tablespoons white sugar

- 1/2 teaspoons cocoa powder
- 1 dash ground cinnamon
- 1 cup boiling water

Directions

- Stir together coconut milk, vanilla extract, sugar, cocoa powder, and cinnamon in a large mug. Add boiling water and stir until thesugar has dissolved.

Vegan Apple Carrot Muffins

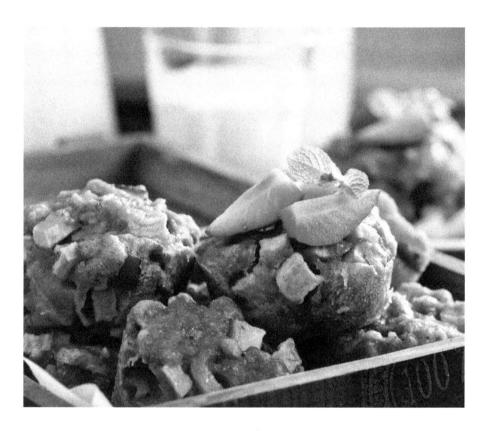

Ingredients

- cup brown sugar

- 1/2 cup white sugar
- 1/2 cups all-purpose flour
- 4 teaspoons baking soda

- 1 teaspoon baking powder

- teaspoons ground cinnamon

- 2 teaspoons salt

- 2 cups finely grated carrots

- 2 large apples - peeled, cored and shredded

- teaspoons egg replacer (dry)

- 1 1/4 cups applesauce

- 1/4 cup vegetable oil

Directions

- Preheat oven to 375 degrees F (190 degrees C). Grease muffincups or line with paper muffin liners.

- In a large bowl combine brown sugar, white sugar, flour, baking soda, baking powder, cinnamon and salt. Stir in carrot and apple;mix well.

- In a small bowl whisk together egg substitute, applesauce and oil.Stir into dry ingredients.

- Spoon batter into prepared pans.

- Bake in preheated oven for 20 minutes. Let muffins cool in pan for5 minutes before removing from pans to cool completely.

Vegan Lentil, Kale, and Red Onion Pasta

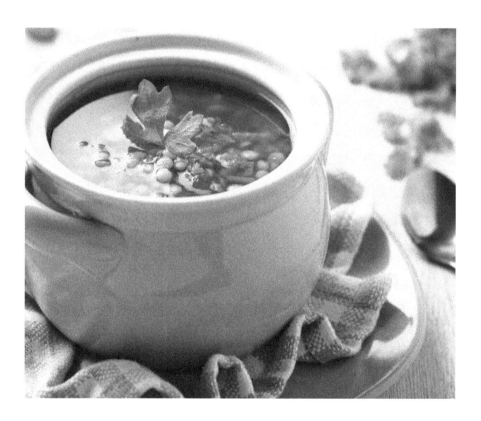

Ingredients

- 2 1/2 cups vegetable broth
- 3/4 cup dry lentils
- 1/2 teaspoon salt1 bay leaf
- 1/4 cup olive oil
- 1 large red onion, chopped
- 1 teaspoon chopped fresh thyme
- 1/2 teaspoon chopped fresh oregano
- 1/2 teaspoon salt

- 1/2 teaspoon black pepper
- 8 ounces vegan sausage, cut into
- 1/4 inch slices (optional)
- 1 bunch kale, stems removed andleaves coarsely chopped
- 1 (12 ounce) package rotini pasta2 tablespoons nutritional yeast (optional)

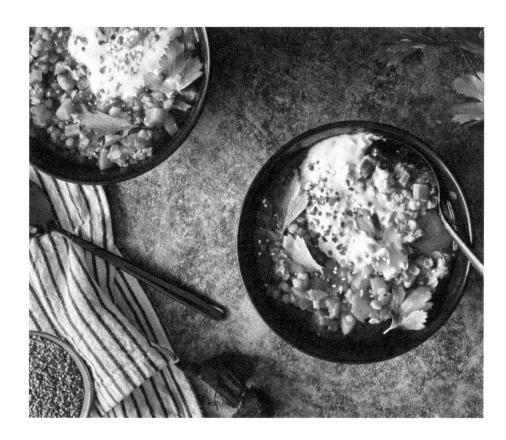

Directions

- Bring the vegetable broth, lentils, 1/2 teaspoon of salt, and bay leaf to a boil in a saucepan over high heat. Reduce heat to medium-low, cover, and cook until the lentils are tender, about 20 minutes. Add additional broth if needed to keep the lentils moist. Discard the bay leaf once done.

- As the lentils simmer, heat the olive oil in a skillet over medium-high heat. Stir in the onion, thyme, oregano, 1/2 teaspoon of salt, and pepper. Cook and stir for 1 minute, then add the sausage. Reduce the heat to medium-low, and cook until the onion has softened, about 10 minutes.

- Meanwhile, bring a large pot of lightly salted water to a boil over high heat. Add the kale and rotini pasta. Cook until the rotini is aldente, about 8 minutes. Remove some of the cooking water, and set aside. Drain the pasta, then return to the pot, and stir in the lentils, and onion mixture. Use the reserved cooking liquid to adjustthe moistness of the dish to your liking. Sprinkle with nutritional yeast to serve.

Vegan Granola

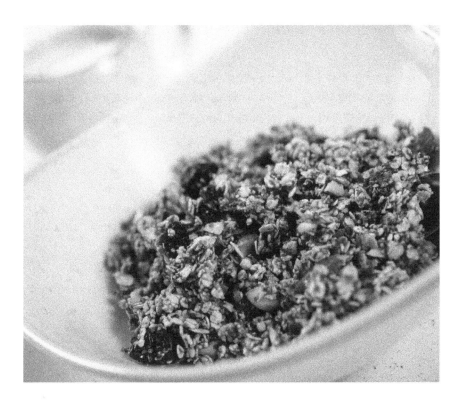

Ingredients

- cooking spray
- 3 cups rolled oats
- 2/3 cup wheat germ
- 1/2 cup slivered almonds
- 1 pinch ground nutmeg
- 1 1/2 teaspoons ground cinnamon
- 1/2 cup apple juice
- 1/2 cup molasses
- 1 teaspoon vanilla extract
- 1 cup dried mixed fruit
- 1 cup quartered dried apricots

Directions

- Preheat oven to 350 degrees F (175 degrees C). Prepare two cookie sheets with cooking spray.

- In a large bowl, combine oats, wheat germ, almonds, cinnamon and nutmeg. In a separate bowl, mix apple juice, molasses and extract. Pour the wet ingredients into the dry ingredients, stirring to coat.
- Spread mixture onto baking sheets.

- Bake for 30 minutes in preheated oven, stirring mixture every 10 to 15 minutes, or until granola has a golden brown color. Let cool. Stir in dried fruit. Store in an airtight container.

Vegan Baked Oatmeal Patties

Ingredients

- cups water
- 4 cups quick cooking oats
- 1/2 onion, chopped
- 1/3 cup vegetable oil
- 1/2 cup spaghetti sauce
- 1/2 cup chopped pecans
- 1/4 cup nutritional yeast
- 2 teaspoons garlic powder1 teaspoon dried basil
- 2 teaspoons onion powder
- 1 teaspoon ground coriander1 teaspoon sage
- 1 teaspoon active dry yeast

Directions

- Preheat oven to 350 degrees F (175 degrees C). Grease a baking sheet.
- Bring water to a boil and stir in oatmeal. Cover and reduce heat tolow. Cook 5 to 10 minutes, or until the oats are cooked and all thewater has been absorbed. Remove from heat and let stand for 5 minutes.
- To the oatmeal add onion, oil, spaghetti sauce, pecans, nutritionalyeast, garlic powder, basil, onion powder, coriander, sage and active yeast. Mix well and form into patties. Place on prepared baking sheet.
- Bake for 15 minutes. Turn patties over and bake another 15minutes.

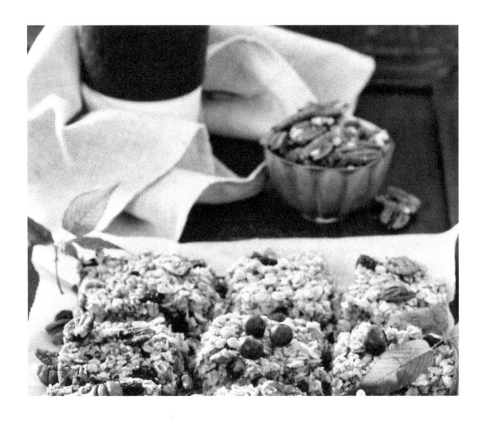

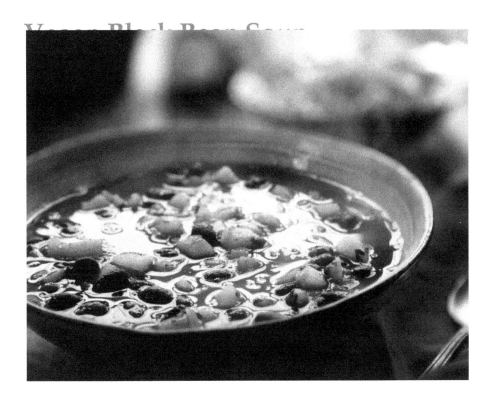

Ingredients

- 1 tablespoon olive oil
- 1 large onion, chopped
- 1 stalk celery, chopped
- 2 carrots, chopped
- cloves garlic, chopped
- 2 tablespoons chili powder
- 1 tablespoon ground cumin
- 1 pinch black pepper
- 4 cups vegetable broth
- 4 (15 ounce) cans black beans
- 1 (15 ounce) can whole kernelcorn
- 1 (14.5 ounce) can crushedtomatoes

Directions

- Heat oil in a large pot over medium-high heat. Saute onion, celery, carrots and garlic for 5 minutes. Season with chili powder, cumin, and black pepper; cook for 1 minute. Stir in vegetable broth, 2 cansof beans, and corn. Bring to a boil.

- Meanwhile, in a food processor or blender, process remaining 2cans beans and tomatoes until smooth. Stir into boiling soup mixture, reduce heat to medium, and simmer for 15 minutes.

Vegan Taco Chili

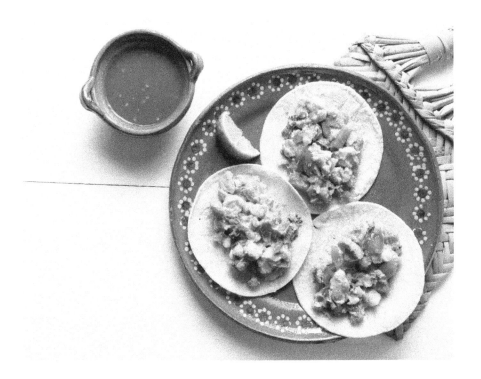

Ingredients

- 1 tablespoon olive oil
- 1 pound sliced fresh mushrooms
- 2 cloves garlic, minced
- 1 small onion, finely chopped
- 2 stalks celery, chopped
- 1 (29 ounce) can tomato sauce
- 1 (6 ounce) can tomato paste
- 3 (15 ounce) cans kidney beans
- 1 (11 ounce) can Mexican-stylecorn

Directions

- Heat the oil in a large skillet. Sautee the mushrooms, garlic, onion and celery until tender. Transfer them to a stock pot or slow cooker.Stir in the tomato sauce, tomato paste, beans and Mexican-style corn. Cook for at least an hour to blend the flavors.
-

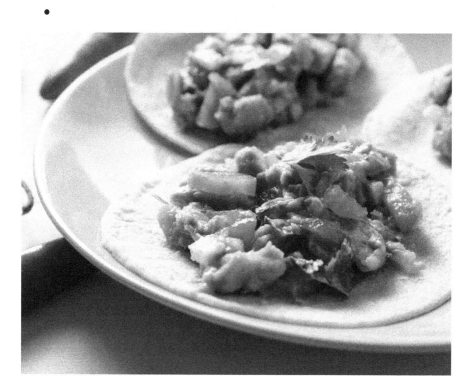

Easy Vegan Whole Grain Pancakes

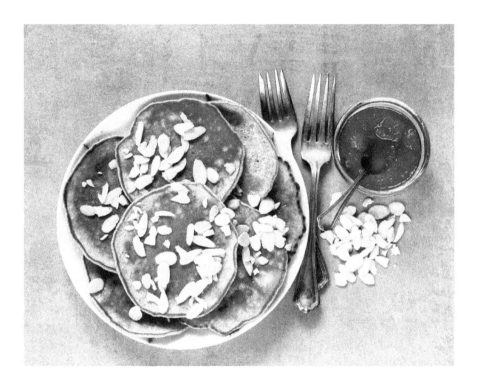

Ingredients

- 1/2 cup whole wheat flour
- 1/2 cup rye flour
- 1 tablespoon soy flour
- 1 tablespoon white sugar
- 1 1/2 teaspoons baking powder
- 1/8 teaspoon salt
- 1/8 teaspoon ground cinnamon(optional)
- 1/2 teaspoon vanilla extract(optional)
- 1/2 cup water 1/2 cup soy milk
- 1/4 cup chopped pecans

Directions

- In a medium bowl, stir together the whole wheat flour, rye flour, soyflour, sugar, baking powder, salt and cinnamon. Make a well in the center, and pour in the vanilla, water and soy milk. Mix until all ofthe dry ingredients have been absorbed, then stir in the pecans.
- Heat a large skillet or griddle iron over medium heat, and coat with cooking spray. Pour about 1/3 cup of batter onto the hot surface, and spread out to 1/4 inch thickness. Cook until bubbles appear onthe surface, then flip and brown on the other side. Serve warm

Vegan Stew

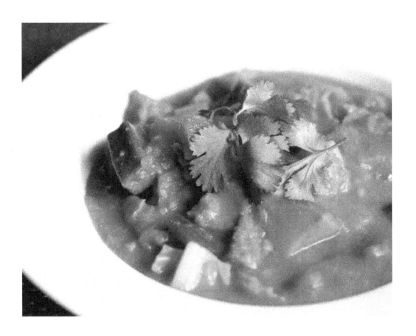

Ingredients

- 1 onion, chopped
- 3 carrots, chopped
- 3 potatoes, chopped
- 1 parsnip, chopped
- 1 turnip, chopped
- 1/4 cup uncooked white rice
- 1 teaspoon ground black pepper1 teaspoon ground cumin
- 1 teaspoon salt 2 1/2 cups water

Directions

- In a large pot over medium-high heat, combine onion, carrots, potatoes, parsnip, turnip, rice, pepper, cumin, salt and water. Boil until vegetables are tender, about 30 minutes, adding more water if necessary.

Vegan Crepes

Ingredients

- 1/2 cup soy milk
- 1/2 cup water
- 1/4 cup melted soy margarine
- 1 tablespoon turbinado sugar
- 2 tablespoons maple syrup
- 1 cup unbleached all-purposeflour
- 1/4 teaspoon salt

Directions

- In a large mixing bowl, blend soy milk, water, 1/4 cup margarine, sugar, syrup, flour, and salt. Cover and chill the mixture for 2 hours.

- Lightly grease a 5 to 6 inch skillet with some soy margarine. Heat the skillet until hot. Pour approximately 3 tablespoons batter into the skillet. Swirl to make the batter cover the skillet's bottom. Cookuntil golden, flip and cook on opposite side.

Vegan Chocolate Cake

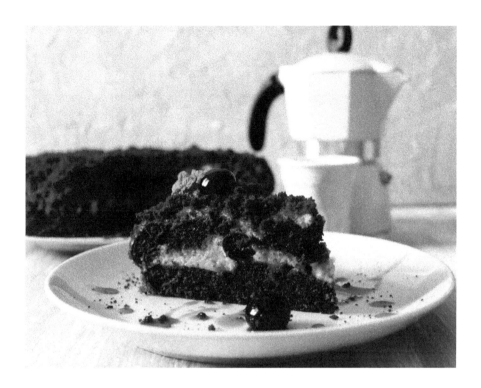

Ingredients

- 1 1/2 cups all-purpose flour1 cup white sugar
- 1/4 cup cocoa powder1 teaspoon baking soda
- 1/2 teaspoon salt
- 1/3 cup vegetable oil
- 1 teaspoon vanilla extract
- 1 teaspoon distilled white vinegar1 cup water

Directions

- Preheat oven to 350 degrees F (175 degrees C). Lightly grease one9x5 inch loaf pan.

- Sift together the flour, sugar, cocoa, baking soda and salt. Add theoil, vanilla, vinegar and water. Mix together until smooth.

- Pour into prepared pan and bake at 350 degrees F (175 degrees C)for 45 minutes. Remove from oven and allow to cool.

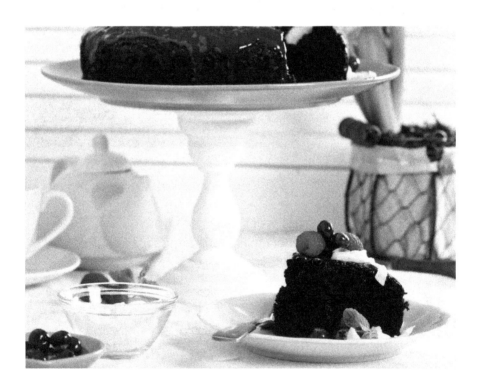

Cyclops Cookies (Vegan)

Ingredients

- 2 cups all-purpose flour
- 1/4 teaspoon ground cinnamon
- 1/4 cup shortening
- 1/4 cup margarine
- 3/4 cup confectioners' sugar
- 1 cup chopped walnuts
- 1 cup semisweet chocolate chips

Directions

- Mix together the flour and cinnamon. In separate large bowl creamtogether shortening, margarine and powdered sugar. Gradually addin the flour/cinnamon mixture. Fold in the chopped nuts.

- Roll out on floured surface to 1/4 inch thickness and cut out cookieswith a 2 inch round cookie cutter. Place 1 inch apart on ungreased cookie sheet.

- Put one single chocolate chip in the center of each cookie. Bake 8
- -10 minutes at 400 degrees F (205 degrees C) until lightly colored.Cool on wire racks.

Vegan Lasagna

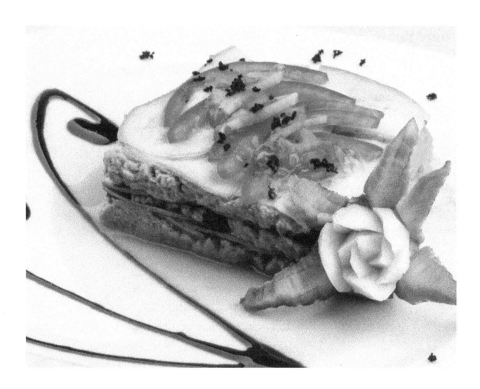

Ingredients

- 2 tablespoons olive oil
- 1 1/2 cups chopped onion
- 3 tablespoons minced garlic4 (14.5 ounce) cans stewed tomatoes
- 1/3 cup tomato paste
- 1/2 cup chopped fresh basil
- 1/2 cup chopped parsley
- 1 teaspoon salt
- teaspoon ground black pepper

- (16 ounce) package lasagnanoodles
- pounds firm tofu

- tablespoons minced garlic1/4 cup chopped fresh basil
- 1/4 cup chopped parsley
- 1/2 teaspoon salt
- ground black pepper to taste 3 (10 ounce) packages frozen chopped spinach, thawed anddrained

Directions

- Make the sauce: In a large, heavy saucepan, over medium heat, heat the olive oil. Place the onions in the saucepan and saute themuntil they are soft, about 5 minutes. Add the garlic; cook 5 minutesmore.

- Place the tomatoes, tomato paste, basil and parsley in the saucepan. Stir well, turn the heat to low and let the sauce simmercovered for 1 hour. Add the salt and pepper.

- While the sauce is cooking bring a large kettle of salted water to aboil. Boil the lasagna noodles for 9 minutes, then drain and rinsewell.

- Preheat the oven to 400 degrees F (200 degrees C).

- Place the tofu blocks in a large bowl. Add the garlic, basil and parsley. Add the salt and pepper, and mash all the ingredients together by squeezing pieces of tofu through your fingers. Mix well.

- Assemble the lasagna: Spread 1 cup of the tomato sauce in the bottom of a 9x13 inch casserole pan. Arrange a single layer of lasagna noodles, sprinkle one-third of the tofu mixture over the noodles. Distribute the spinach evenly over the tofu. Next ladle 1 1/2 cups tomato sauce over the tofu, and top it with another layer of the noodles. Then sprinkle another 1/3 of the tofu mixture over the noodles, top the tofu with 1 1/2 cups tomato sauce, and place a final layer of noodles over the tomato sauce. Finally, top the noodles with the final 1/3 of the tofu, and spread the remaining tomato sauce over everything.

- Cover the pan with foil and bake the lasagna for 30 minutes. Serve hot and enjoy.

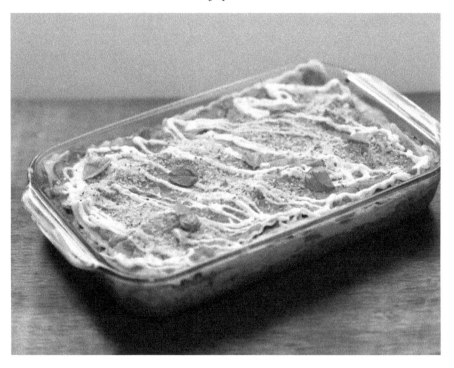

Easy Vegan Peanut Butter Fudge

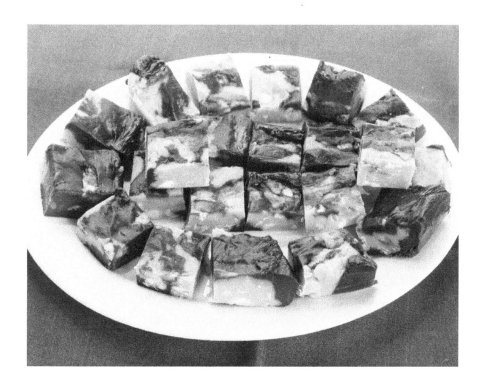

Ingredients

- 3/4 cup vegan margarine1 cup peanut butter
- 3 2/3 cups confectioners' sugar

Directions

- Lightly grease a 9x9 inch baking dish.

- In a saucepan over low heat, melt margarine. Remove from heat and stir in peanut butter until smooth. Stir in confectioners' sugar, alittle at a time, until well blended. Pat into prepared pan and chill until firm. Cut into squares.

Yummy Vegan Chocolate Pudding

Ingredients

- 2 tablespoons cornstarch1 cup soy milk
- 1 cup soy creamer
- 1/2 cup white sugar
- 3 tablespoons egg replacer (dry)3 ounces semisweet chocolate, chopped
- 2 teaspoons vanilla extract

Directions

- In a medium saucepan combine cornstarch, soy milk and soy creamer; stir to dissolve cornstarch. Place on medium heat and stirin sugar. Cook, whisking frequently, until mixture comes to a low boil; remove from heat.

- In a small bowl whisk egg replacer with 1/4 cup of hot milk mixture; return to pan with remaining milk mixture. Cook over medium heat for 3 to 4 minutes, until thick, but not boiling.

- Place the chocolate in a medium bowl and pour in the hot milkmixture. Let stand for 30 seconds, then stir until melted and smooth. Cool for 10 to 15 minutes, then stir in vanilla.

- Pour into ramekins or custard cups. Cover with plastic wrap and letcool at room temperature. Refrigerate for 3 hours, or overnight before serving.

Fluffy Vegan Pancakes

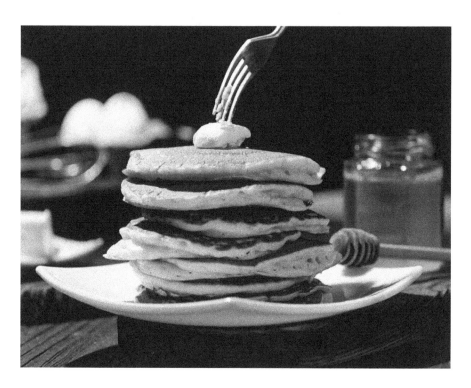

Ingredients

- 1 1/4 cups all-purpose flour
- 1 tablespoon baking powder
- 1/2 teaspoon fine sea salt
- 1/4 cup pureed extra-firm tofu1 cup soy milk
- 1 tablespoon canola oil1/2 cup water

Directions

- Whisk together the flour, baking powder, and sea salt; set aside.

- Whisk together the tofu, soy milk, canola oil, and water. Graduallywhisk the flour mixture into the tofu mixture, making sure to beat out all lumps between additions.

- Heat a lightly oiled griddle over medium-high heat. Drop batter bylarge spoonfuls onto the griddle, and cook until lightly browned onthe bottom. Flip, and cook until lightly browned on the other side. Repeat with remaining batter.

-

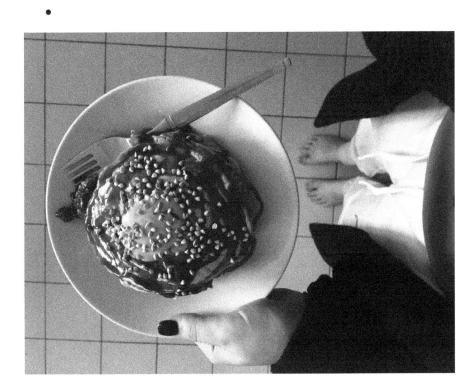

Vegan Avocado Dip

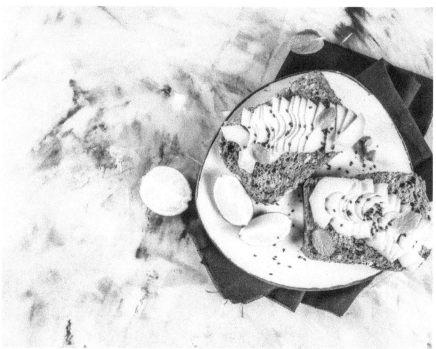

Ingredients

- 2 avocados - peeled, pitted anddiced
- 1 (19 ounce) can black beans,drained and rinsed
- 1 (11 ounce) can whole kernelcorn, drained
- 1 medium onion, minced3/4 cup salsa
- 1 tablespoon chopped freshcilantro
- 1 tablespoon lemon juice
- 2 tablespoons chili powdersalt and pepper to taste

Directions

- In a bowl, mix the avocados, black beans, corn, onion, salsa, cilantro, and lemon juice. Season with chili powder, salt, and pepper.

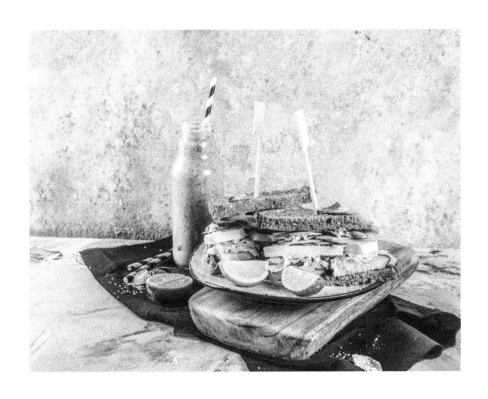

Vegan Curried Rice

Ingredients

- 2 tablespoons olive oil
- 1 tablespoon minced garlicblack pepper to taste
- 1 tablespoon ground cumin, or totaste
- 1 tablespoon ground currypowder, or to taste
- 1 tablespoon chili powder, or totaste
- 1 cube vegetable bouillon1 cup water
- 1 tablespoon soy sauce
- 1 cup uncooked white rice

Directions

- Heat olive oil in a medium saucepan over low heat. Sweat the garlic; when the garlic becomes aromatic, slowly stir in pepper, cumin, curry powder and chili powder. When spices begin to fryand become fragrant, stir in the bouillon cube and a little water.

- Increase heat to high and add the rest of the water and the soy sauce. Just before the mixture comes to a boil, stir in rice. Bring to a rolling boil; reduce heat to low, cover, and simmer 15 to 20 minutes, or until all liquid is absorbed.

- Remove from heat and let stand 5 minutes.

Vegan-Friendly Falafel

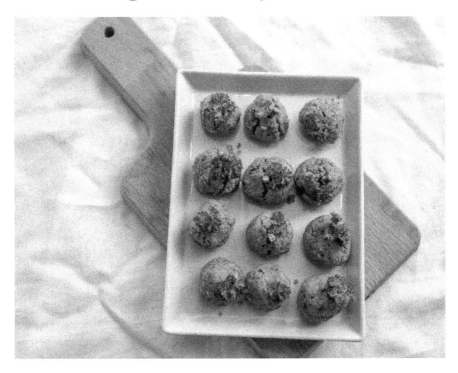

Ingredients

- 1 pound dry garbanzo beans1 onion, quartered
- 1 potato, peeled and quartered
- 4 cloves garlic, minced
- 1/2 cup cilantro leaves, chopped
- 1 teaspoon ground coriander
- 1 teaspoon ground cumin
- 2 teaspoons salt
- 1/2 teaspoon ground blackpepper
- 1/2 teaspoon cayenne pepper2 teaspoons fresh lemon juice
  1 tablespoon olive oil

- tablespoon all-purpose flour
- 2 teaspoons baking soda

- cups canola oil

Directions

- Rinse the garbanzo beans under cold water and discard any bad ones. Place in a large pot, and cover with water. Let soak 24 hours, and rinse again.

- Place the garbanzo beans, onion, and potato in the bowl of a foodprocessor. Cover, and process until finely chopped. Leaving about1 cup of the garbanzo bean mixture in the food processor bowl, pour the rest into a mixing bowl. Add the garlic, cilantro, coriander,cumin, salt, pepper, and cayenne pepper to the garbanzo bean mixture in the food processor bowl; process on low to blend thoroughly. Return the reserved garbanzo bean mixture to the food processor bowl, and add the lemon juice, and olive oil; process onlow into a coarse meal. Cover, and refrigerate 2 hours.

- Stir the baking soda into the garbanzo bean mixture until evenlyblended. Using damp hands, form the mixture into 1 1/2 inch diameter balls.

- Pour the canola oil into a wok 1 to 2 inches deep, and heat over medium-high heat. Cook the falafel balls, turning so all sides are evenly browned, about 5 minutes. Remove falafel from oil, and drainon paper towels. Repeat to cook remaining falafel balls.

Simple Vegan Icing

Ingredients

- 1/2 cup vegetable shortening
- 4 cups confectioners' sugar
- 5 tablespoons soy milk
- 1/4 teaspoon vanilla extract

Directions

- Beat the shortening and confectioners' sugar together until the shortening has been incorporated, and the mixture is clumpy. Pourin the soy milk and vanilla extract; beat until smooth.

Penne with Vegan Arrabbiata Sauce

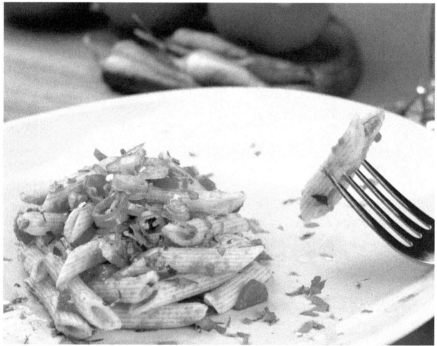

Ingredients

- 1 cup extra virgin olive oil
- 7 cloves garlic, minced
- 7 (28 ounce) cans crushedtomatoes
- 2 1/2 teaspoons crushed redpepper flakes
- 2 bay leaves
- 10 leaves fresh basil

Directions

- Bring a large pot of lightly salted water to a boil. Add pasta andcook for 8 to 10 minutes or until al dente; drain.

- Heat olive oil, and cook garlic just until softened. Add remainingingredients. Simmer over low heat and cook at least 3 hours.

- Add the cooked penne pasta and let sit at least 5 minutes before stirring and serving. Sprinkle with 1/2 cup grated Romano or parmesan cheese, if desired.

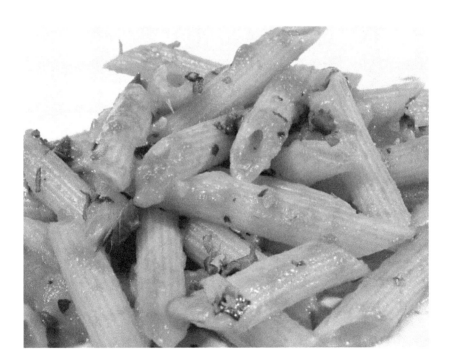

Kingman's Vegan Zucchini Bread

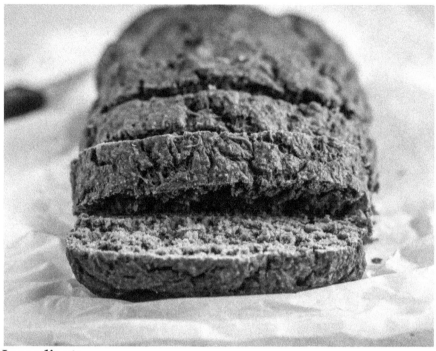

Ingredients

- 3 cups all-purpose flour
- 3 tablespoons flax seeds(optional)
- teaspoon salt

- teaspoon baking soda
- teaspoons ground cinnamon
- 1/2 teaspoon baking powder
- 1/2 teaspoon arrowroot powder(optional)
- cup unsweetened applesauce1 cup white sugar

- cup packed brown sugar
- 3/4 cup vegetable oil
- teaspoons vanilla extract

- 1/2 cups shredded zucchini

Directions

- Preheat oven to 325 degrees F (165 degrees C). Grease and flourtwo 9x5 inch loaf pans. Whisk together the flour, flax seeds, salt,baking soda, cinnamon, baking powder, and arrowroot in a bowluntil evenly blended; set aside.

- Whisk together the applesauce, white sugar, brown sugar, vegetable oil, and vanilla extract in a bowl until smooth. Fold in the flour mixture and shredded zucchini until moistened. Divide the batter between the prepared loaf pans.

- Bake in the preheated oven until a toothpick inserted into the center comes out clean, about 70 minutes. Cool in the pans for 10 minutesbefore removing to cool completely on a wire rack.

Vegan Red Lentil Soup

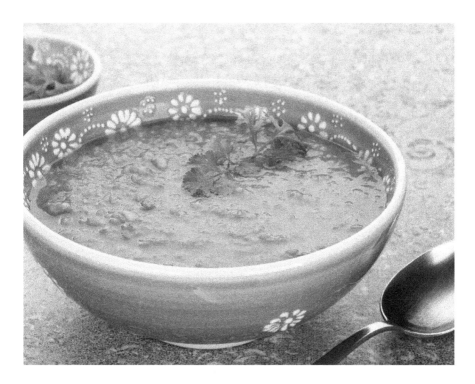

Ingredients

- 1 tablespoon peanut oil1 small onion, chopped
- 1 tablespoon minced fresh gingerroot
- clove garlic, chopped
- 1 pinch fenugreek seeds1 cup dry red lentils

- cup butternut squash - peeled,seeded, and cubed
- 1/3 cup finely chopped freshcilantro

- cups water
- 1/2 (14 ounce) can coconut milk2 tablespoons tomato paste
- 1 teaspoon curry powder1 pinch cayenne pepper
- 1 pinch ground nutmeg salt and pepper to taste

Directions

- Heat the oil in a large pot over medium heat, and cook the onion,ginger, garlic, and fenugreek until onion is tender.

- Mix the lentils, squash, and cilantro into the pot. Stir in the water, coconut milk, and tomato paste. Season with curry powder, cayenne pepper, nutmeg, salt, and pepper. Bring to a boil, reduceheat to low, and simmer 30 minutes, or until lentils and squash aretender.

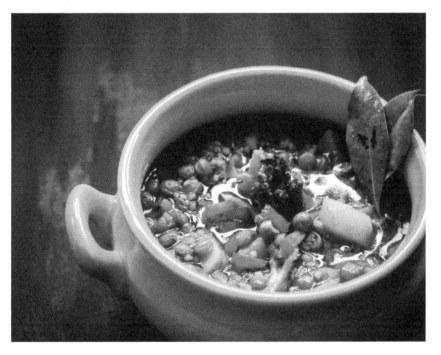

Vegan Lemon Poppy Scones

Ingredients

- 2 cups all-purpose flour
- 3/4 cup white sugar
- 4 teaspoons baking powder
- 1/2 teaspoon salt
- 3/4 cup margarine
- 1 lemon, zested and juiced2 tablespoons poppy seeds
  1/2 cup soy milk
- 1/2 cup water

Directions

- Preheat the oven to 400 degrees F (200 degrees C). Grease abaking sheet.

- Sift the flour, sugar, baking powder and salt into a large bowl. Cut in margarine until the mixture is the consistency of large grains of sand. I like to use my hands to rub the margarine into the flour. Stir in poppy seeds, lemon zest and lemon juice. Combine the soy milk and water, and gradually stir into the dry ingredients until the batter is moistened, but still thick like biscuit dough. You may not need all of the liquid.

- Spoon 1/4 cup sized plops of batter onto the greased baking sheetso they are about 3 inches apart.

- Bake for 10 to 15 minutes the preheated oven, until golden.

Bold Vegan Chili

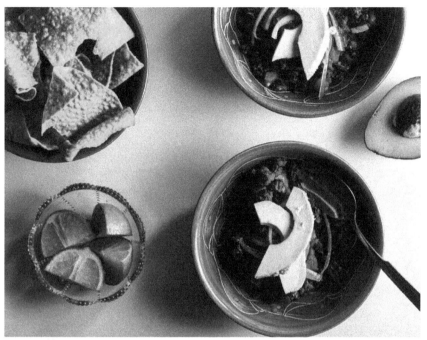

Ingredients

- 1 (12 ounce) package vegetarianburger crumbles
- 3 (15.25 ounce) cans kidneybeans

- large red onion, chopped
- 4 stalks celery, diced
- red bell peppers, chopped
- 4 bay leaves
- 2 tablespoons hot chili powder3 tablespoons molasses
- 1 cube vegetable bouillon
- 1 tablespoon chopped freshcilantro
- 1 teaspoon hot pepper saucesalt and pepper to taste
- 1 cup water
- 3 tablespoons all-purpose flour1 cup hot water

Directions

- In a slow cooker combine vegetarian crumbles, kidney beans, onion, celery, bell pepper, bay leaves, chili powder, molasses, bouillon, cilantro, hot sauce, salt, pepper and 1 cup water. Cook onhigh for 3 hours.

-

- Dissolve flour in 1 cup hot water. Pour into chili and cook 1 morehour.

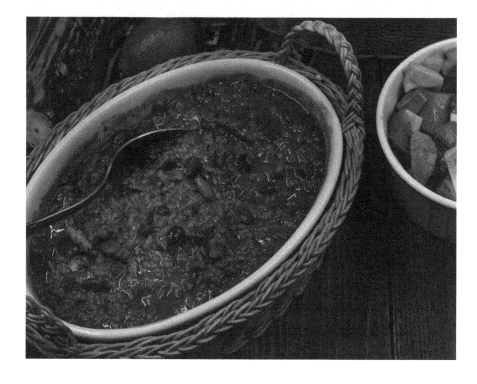

Vegan Hot and Sour Soup

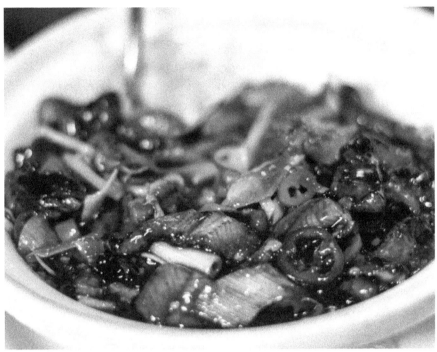

Ingredients

- 1 ounce dried wood earmushrooms
- 4 dried shiitake mushrooms
- 12 dried tiger lily buds
- 2 cups hot water
- 1/3 ounce bamboo fungus3 tablespoons soy sauce
- 5 tablespoons rice vinegar
- 1/4 cup cornstarch
- 1 (8 ounce) container firm tofu, cutinto
- 1/4 inch strips
- 1 quart vegetable broth
- 1/4 teaspoon crushed red pepperflakes
- 1/2 teaspoon ground blackpepper
- 3/4 teaspoon ground whitepepper

- 1/2 tablespoon chili oil 1/2 tablespoon sesame oil1 green onion, sliced
- 1 cup Chinese dried mushrooms

Directions

- In a small bowl, place wood mushrooms, shiitake mushrooms, and lily buds in 1 1/2 cups hot water. Soak 20 minutes, until rehydrated.Drain, reserving liquid. Trim stems from the mushrooms, and cut into thin strips. Cut the lily buds in half.

- In a separate small bowl, soak bamboo fungus in 1/4 cup lightlysalted hot water. Soak about 20 minutes, until rehydrated. Drain,and mince.

- In a third small bowl, blend soy sauce, rice vinegar, and 1 tablespoon cornstarch. Place 1/2 the tofu strips into the mixture.

- In a medium saucepan, mix the reserved mushroom and lily bud liquid with the vegetable broth. Bring to a boil, and stir in the woodmushrooms, shiitake mushrooms, and lily buds. Reduce heat, and simmer 3 to 5 minutes. Season with red pepper, black pepper, andwhite pepper.

- In a small bowl, mix remaining cornstarch and remaining water. Stirinto the broth mixture until thickened.

- Mix soy sauce mixture and remaining tofu strips into the saucepan.Return to boil, and stir in the bamboo fungus, chili oil, and sesame oil. Garnish with green onion to serve.

Vegan Banana Blueberry Muffins

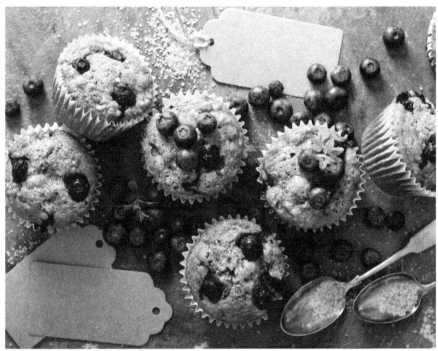

Ingredients

- 2 very ripe bananas, mashed
- 1/2 cup white sugar
- 1/2 teaspoon baking powder
- 1/2 teaspoon salt
- 3/4 cup all-purpose flour
- 1/2 cup whole wheat pastry flour
- 1.1/2 teaspoons egg replacer (dry)2 tablespoons water
- 1/2 cup blueberries

Directions

Preheat oven to 350 degrees F (175 degrees C). Grease muffincups or line with paper muffin liners.

In a large bowl combine mashed bananas, sugar, baking powder,salt and flours; mix until smooth. In a small bowl or cup combineegg replacer and water; stir into banana mixture. Fold in blueberries.

Spoon batter evenly, about 1/4 cup each, into muffin cups.

Bake in preheated oven for 20 to 25 minutes, or until golden brown.

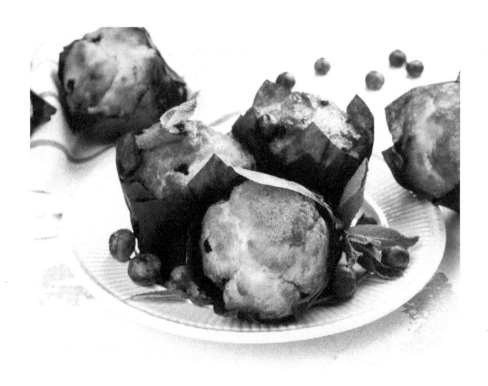

Spicy Vegan Potato Curry

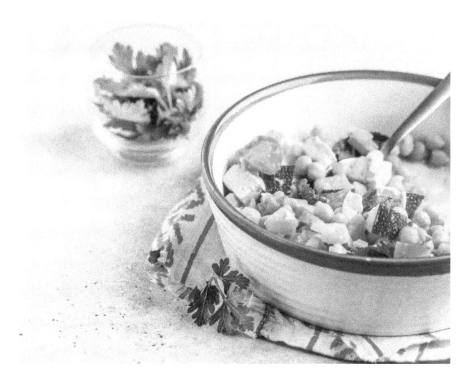

Ingredients

- 4 potatoes, peeled and cubed
- 2 tablespoons vegetable oil

- yellow onion, diced
- 3 cloves garlic, minced
- teaspoons ground cumin
- 1.1/2 teaspoons cayenne pepper
- 4 teaspoons curry powder
- 4 teaspoons garam masala

- (1 inch) piece fresh ginger root,peeled and minced
- teaspoons salt

- 1 (14.5 ounce) can diced tomatoes
- 1 (15 ounce) can garbanzo beans(chickpeas), rinsed and drained
- 1 (15 ounce) can peas, drained
- 1 (14 ounce) can coconut milk

Directions

- Place potatoes into a large pot and cover with salted water. Bring toa boil over high heat, then reduce heat to medium-low, cover, and simmer until just tender, about 15 minutes. Drain and allow to steamdry for a minute or two.

- Meanwhile, heat the vegetable oil in a large skillet over medium heat. Stir in the onion and garlic; cook and stir until the onion has softened and turned translucent, about 5 minutes. Season with cumin, cayenne pepper, curry powder, garam masala, ginger, andsalt; cook for 2 minutes more. Add the tomatoes, garbanzo beans,peas, and potatoes. Pour in the coconut milk, and bring to a simmer. Simmer 5 to 10 minutes before serving.

Vegan Brownies

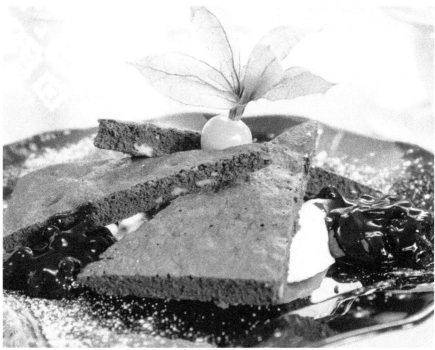

Ingredients

- 2 cups unbleached all-purposeflour
- 2 cups white sugar
- 3/4 cup unsweetened cocoapowder
- 1 teaspoon baking powder
- 1 teaspoon salt
- 1 cup water
- 1 cup vegetable oil
- 1 teaspoon vanilla extract

Directions

- Preheat the oven to 350 degrees F (175 degrees C).

- In a large bowl, stir together the flour, sugar, cocoa powder, bakingpowder and salt. Pour in water, vegetable oil and vanilla; mix until well blended. Spread evenly in a 9x13 inch baking pan.

- Bake for 25 to 30 minutes in the preheated oven, until the top is nolonger shiny. Let cool for at least 10 minutes before cutting into squares.

Best Vegan Pancakes

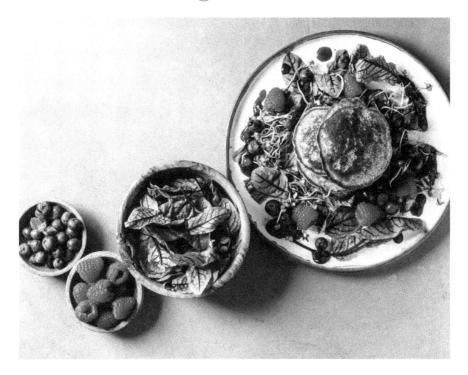

Ingredients

- 4 cups self-rising flour
- 1 tablespoon white sugar
- 1 tablespoon custard powder2 cups soy milk

Directions

- In a large bowl, stir together the flour, sugar and custard powder.Mix in the soy milk with a whisk so there are no lumps.
- Heat a griddle over medium heat, and coat with nonstick cooking spray. Spoon batter onto the surface, and cook until bubbles begin to form on the surface. Flip with a spatula and cook on the other side until golden.

Vegan Corn Bread

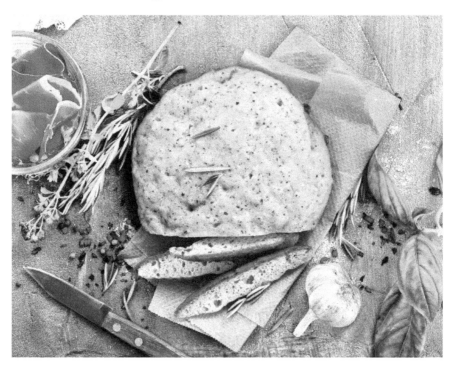

Ingredients

- 1 cup all-purpose flour1 cup cornmeal
- 1/4 cup turbinado sugar
- 1 tablespoon baking powder
- 1 teaspoon salt
- 1 cup sweetened, plain soy milk
- 1/3 cup vegetable oil
- 1/4 cup soft silken tofu

Directions

- Preheat an oven to 400 degrees F (200 degrees C). Grease a 7 inch square baking pan. Whisk together the flour, cornmeal, sugar, baking powder, and salt in a mixing bowl; set aside.

- Place the soy milk, oil, and tofu into a blender. Cover, and puree until smooth. Make a well in the center of the cornmeal mixture. Pour the pureed tofu into the well, then stir in the cornmeal mixture until just moistened. Pour the batter into the prepared baking pan.

- Bake in the preheated oven until a toothpick inserted into the centercomes out clean, 20 to 25 minutes. Cut into 9 pieces, and serve warm.

Quick Vegan Spaghetti Sauce

Ingredients

- 1 (29 ounce) can tomato sauce
- 1 (6 ounce) can sliced mushrooms, drained
- 1/2 cup chopped celery1/4 cup diced red onion
- 1/4 cup raisins
- 1/4 cup chopped walnuts1 tomato, quartered
- 1 large orange, quartered 1 tablespoon minced garlic

Directions

- In a large, heavy saucepan combine tomato sauce, mushrooms, celery, red onion, raisins, walnuts, tomato, orange and garlic. Cook on medium-high until vegetables are tender, about 30 minutes.

Vegan Corn Muffins

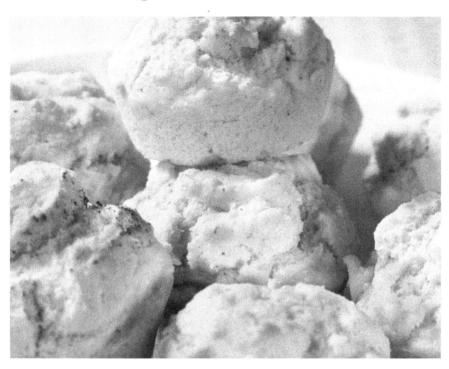

Ingredients

- 1.1/2 teaspoons egg replacer (dry)
- 2 tablespoons water

- 1 cup yellow cornmeal
- 1/2 cup all-purpose flour
- teaspoons baking powder
- 2 tablespoons white sugar
- 2 tablespoons vegetable oil1 cup water
- 1/2 teaspoon salt

Directions

- Preheat oven to 450 degrees F (230 degrees C). Grease six muffincups or line with paper muffin liners.

- In a small bowl, beat together egg replacer and water. In a separatebowl, combine cornmeal, flour, baking powder, sugar and salt. Addegg mixture, oil and water; stir until smooth. Spoon batter into prepared muffin tins using approximately 1/2 cup for each muffin.

- Bake in pre-heated oven for 10 to 15 minutes, until a toothpickinserted into the center of a muffin comes out clean.

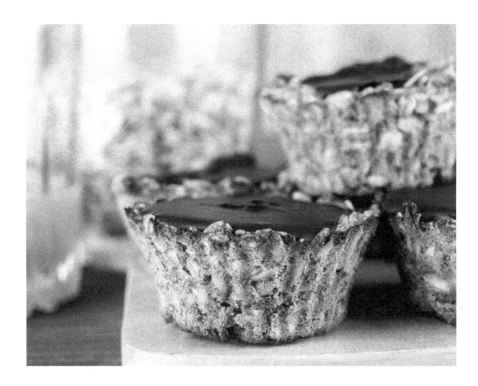

Vegan Potatoes au Gratin

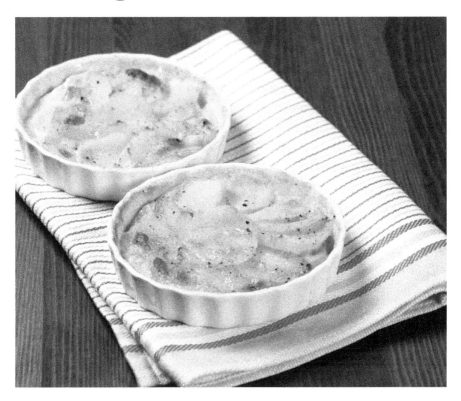

Ingredients

- 1. 1/2 teaspoons egg replacer (dry)
- 2 tablespoons water
- cup yellow cornmeal
- 1/2 cup all-purpose flour
- teaspoons baking powder
- 2 tablespoons white sugar
- 2 tablespoons vegetable oil
- 1 cup water
- 1/2 teaspoon salt

Directions

- Preheat oven to 450 degrees F (230 degrees C). Grease six muffincups or line with paper muffin liners.

- In a small bowl, beat together egg replacer and water. In a separatebowl, combine cornmeal, flour, baking powder, sugar and salt. Addegg mixture, oil and water; stir until smooth. Spoon batter into prepared muffin tins using approximately 1/2 cup for each muffin.

- Bake in pre-heated oven for 10 to 15 minutes, until a toothpickinserted into the center of a muffin comes out clean.

Vegan Split Pea Soup II

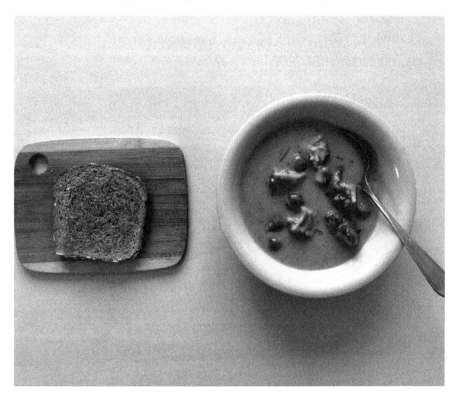

Ingredients

- 1 tablespoon extra virgin olive oil
- 1 carrot, chopped
- 1 stalk celery, chopped
- 1 small onion, chopped
- 1 teaspoon curry powder 1 cup yellow split peas
- 4 cups water
- 1 teaspoon salt

Directions

- Heat olive oil in a large saucepan. Sautee carrot, onion, celery andcurry for about 5 minutes. Add the water, peas and salt. Simmer,stirring occasionally, for 45 to 50 minutes, or until very thick.

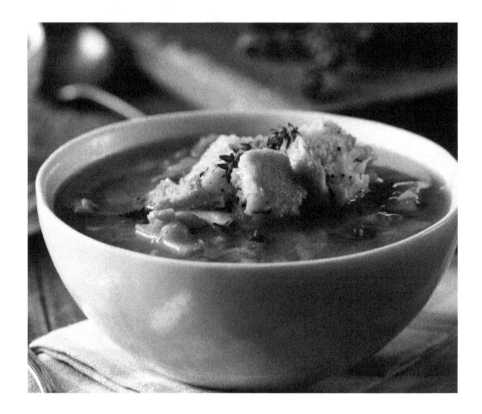

Vegan-Friendly Caramel Buttercream

Ingredients

- 1/2 cup vegan margarine
- 1 cup brown sugar, not packed
- 1/4 cup soy milk
- 1 teaspoon vanilla extract
- 1/2 cup shortening
- 5 cups confectioners' sugar

Directions

- Stir the margarine and brown sugar together in a pan. Bring to a boil over medium-high heat, stirring constantly, and cook for 1 minute until dark brown. Remove from heat, and whisk in the soy milk and vanilla extract until smooth.

- Beat the shortening together with 2 cups confectioners' sugar in a mixing bowl until well blended. Continue beating, and gradually add the brown sugar mixture, alternating with the remaining confectioners' sugar.

Vegan Bean Taco Filling

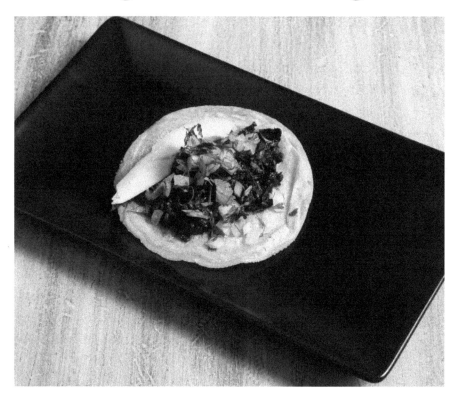

Ingredients

- tablespoon olive oil 1 onion, diced
- cloves garlic, minced
- 1 bell pepper, chopped
- 2 (14.5 ounce) cans black beans, rinsed, drained, and mashed
- 2 tablespoons yellow cornmeal
- 1. 1/2 tablespoons cumin
- 1 teaspoon paprika
- 1 teaspoon cayenne pepper
- 1 teaspoon chili powder
- 1 cup salsa

Directions

- Heat olive oil in a medium skillet over medium heat. Stir in onion, garlic, and bell pepper; cook until tender. Stir in mashed beans. Add the cornmeal. Mix in cumin, paprika, cayenne, chili powder, and salsa. Cover, and cook 5 minutes.

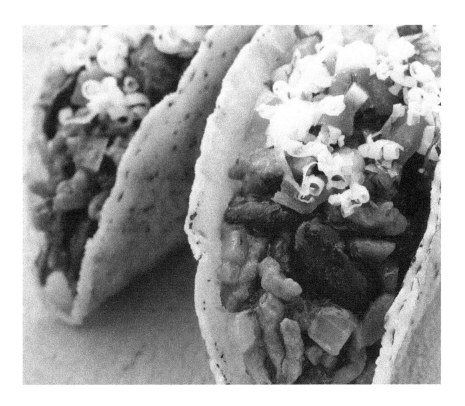

Vegan Split Pea Soup I

Ingredients

- 1 tablespoon vegetable oil 1 onion, chopped
- 1 bay leaf
- 3 cloves garlic, minced
- 2 cups dried split peas
- 1/2 cup barley
- 1. 1/2 teaspoons salt
- 7. 1/2 cups water
- 3 carrots, chopped
- 3 stalks celery, chopped
- 3 potatoes, diced
- 1/2 cup chopped parsley
- 1/2 teaspoon dried basil
- 1/2 teaspoon dried thyme
- 1/2 teaspoon ground black pepper

Directions

- In a large pot over medium high heat, saute the oil, onion, bay leaf and garlic for 5 minutes, or until onions are translucent. Add the peas, barley, salt and water. Bring to a boil and reduce heat to low. Simmer for 2 hours, stirring occasionally.

- Add the carrots, celery, potatoes, parsley, basil, thyme and ground black pepper. Simmer for another hour, or until the peas and vegetables are tender.

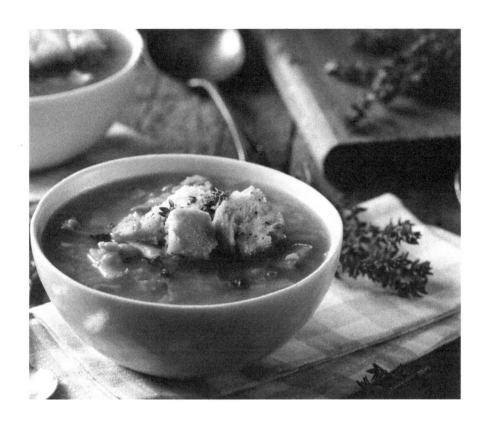

Vegan Agave Cornbread Muffins

Ingredients

- 1/2 cup cornmeal
- 1/2 cup whole-wheat pastry flour
- 1/2 teaspoon baking soda
- 1/2 teaspoon salt 1/2 cup applesauce
- 1/2 cup soy milk
- 1/4 cup agave nectar
- 2 tablespoons canola oil

Directions

- Preheat oven to 325 degrees F (165 degrees C). Lightly grease a muffin pan.

- Combine the cornmeal, flour, baking soda, and salt in a large bowl; stir in the applesauce, soy milk, and agave nectar. Slowly add the oil while stirring. Pour the mixture into the muffin pan.

- Bake in the preheated oven until a toothpick or small knife inserted in the crown of a muffin comes out clean, 15 to 20 minutes.

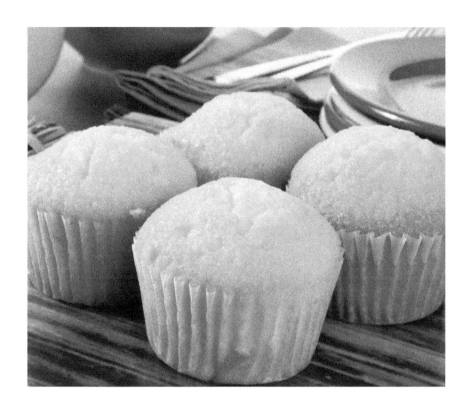

Vegan Cupcakes

Ingredients

- tablespoon apple cider vinegar

- 1. 1/2 cups almond milk
- cups all-purpose flour
- 1 cup white sugar
- 2 teaspoons baking powder
- 1/2 teaspoon baking soda
- 1/2 teaspoon salt
- 1/2 cup coconut oil, warmed until liquid
- 1 1/4 teaspoons vanilla extract

Directions

- Preheat oven to 350 degrees F (175 degrees C). Grease two 12 cupmuffin pans or line with 18 paper baking cups.

- Measure the apple cider vinegar into a 2 cup measuring cup. Fill with almond milk to make 1 1/2 cups. Let stand until curdled, about5 minutes. In a large bowl, Whisk together the flour, sugar, bakingpowder, baking soda and salt. In a separate bowl, whisk together the almond milk mixture, coconut oil and vanilla. Pour the wet ingredients into the dry ingredients and stir just until blended.

- Spoon the batter into the prepared cups, dividing evenly.

- Bake in the preheated oven until the tops spring back when lightlypressed, 15 to 20 minutes. Cool in the pan set over a wire rack.

- When cool, arrange the cupcakes on a serving platter. Frost withdesired frosting.

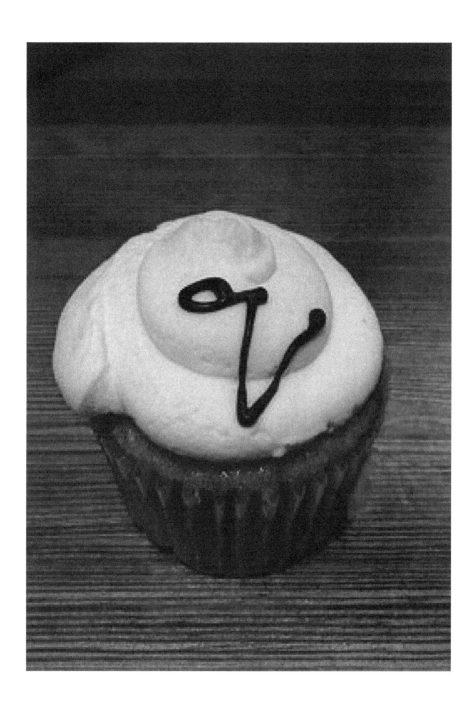

Spicy Thai Vegan Burger

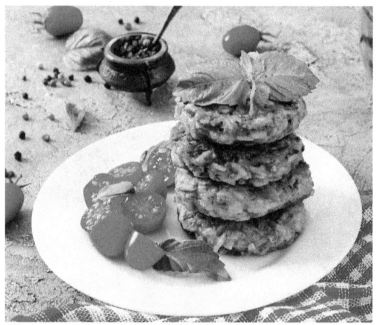

Ingredients

- cup fresh pea pods
- 1/2 cup shredded carrots
- 1/2 cup quartered cherry tomatoes
- 1/3 cup sliced green onions

- tablespoons slivered fresh Thai basil or fresh basil
- 1/4 cup unsweetened light coconut milk or unsweetened coconut milk*
- 1 tablespoon lime juice
- 1/2 teaspoon toasted sesame oil or sesame seeds, toasted
- 1/4 teaspoon crushed red pepper 4 Morningstar FarmsB® GrillersB® Vegan Veggie Burgers 1 (9-inch) focaccia, cut into fourths and horizontally spli

Directions

- Lengthwise cut pea pods into slivers. In medium bowl toss together pea pods, carrots, tomatoes, green onions and basil. Set aside. In small bowl whisk together coconut milk, lime juice, sesame oil and red pepper. Drizzle over vegetables. Toss to coat.

- Cook vegan veggie burgers according to package directions. Serve hot burgers in focaccia, topped with vegetable mixture.

- ON THE GRILL: Preheat grill. Use a food thermometer to be sure patties reach minimum internal temperature of 160 degrees F.

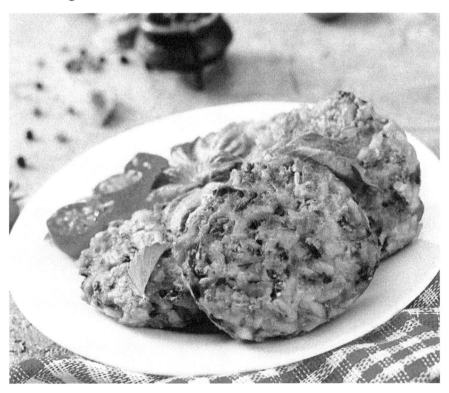

Vegan Fajitas

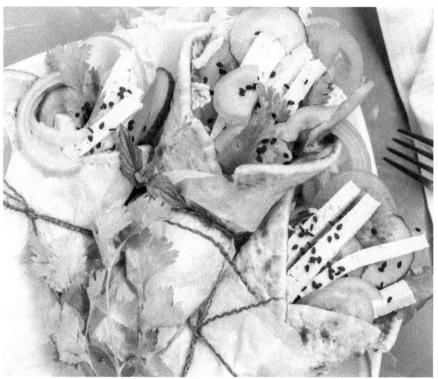

Ingredients

- 1/4 cup olive oil
- 1/4 cup red wine vinegar 1 teaspoon dried oregano 1 teaspoon chili powder garlic salt to taste
- salt and pepper to taste 1 teaspoon white sugar
- 2 small zucchini, julienned
- 2 medium small yellow squash, julienned
- 1 large onion, sliced
- green bell pepper, cut into thin strips
- red bell pepper, cut into thin strips

- tablespoons olive oil
- 1 (8.75 ounce) can whole kernel corn, drained
- 1 (15 ounce) can black beans, drained

Directions

- In a large bowl combine olive oil, vinegar, oregano, chili powder, garlic salt, salt, pepper and sugar. To the marinade add the zucchini, yellow squash, onion, green pepper and red pepper.

- Marinate vegetables in the refrigerator for at least 30 minutes, but not more than 24 hours.

- Heat oil in a large skillet over medium-high heat. Drain the vegetables and saute until tender, about 10 to 15 minutes. Stir in the corn and beans; increase the heat to high for 5 minutes, to brown vegetables.

Vegan Gelatin

Ingredients

- 1/2 teaspoon cornstarch
- 1 teaspoon water
- 2 cups cherry juice or strawberry
- 1 teaspoon agar-agar

Directions

- Dissolve the cornstarch in the water in a small cup or bowl and set aside. In a saucepan, combine 1 1/2 cups of cherry juice and agar- agar powder. Let stand for 5 minutes to soften. Set heat to medium- high and bring to a simmer. Simmer for 1 minute.

- Remove from the heat and stir in the remaining juice along with the cornstarch mixture until no longer cloudy. Pour into small serving cups and refrigerate for 4 hours before serving.

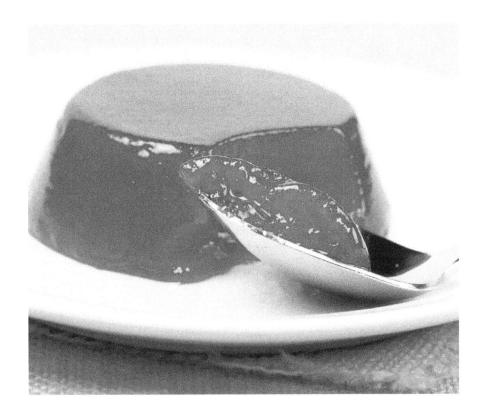

Vegan Cheesecake

Ingredients

- 1 (12 ounce) package soft tofu
- 1/2 cup soy milk
- 1/2 cup white sugar
- 1 tablespoon vanilla extract 1/4 cup maple syrup
- 1 (9 inch) prepared graham cracker crust

Directions

- Preheat oven to 350 degrees F (175 degrees C).

- In a blender, combine the tofu, soy milk, sugar, vanilla extractand maple syrup. Blend until smooth and pour into pie crust.

- Bake at 350 degrees F (175 degrees C) for 30 minutes. Remove from oven and allow to cool; refrigerate until chilled.

Vegan Borscht

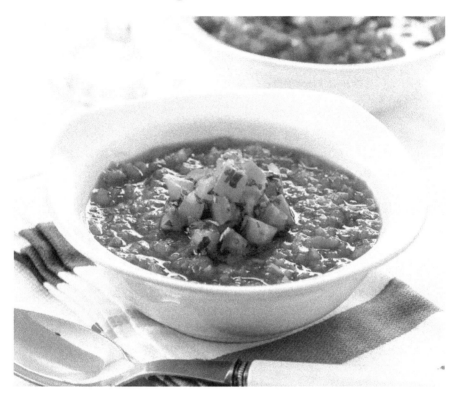

Ingredients

- 1 tablespoon olive oil
- 3 cloves garlic, minced
- 1 onion, chopped
- 3 tablespoons olive oil
- 2 stalks celery, chopped (optional)
- 2 carrots, finely chopped
- 1 green bell pepper, chopped
- 3 beets, including greens, diced
- 1 (16 ounce) can whole peeled tomatoes
- 1/2 cup canned peeled and diced tomatoes
- 2 potatoes, quartered

- 1 cup shredded Swiss chard
- 2 cups vegetable broth
- 4 cups water
- 2 tablespoons dried dill weed salt and freshly ground black pepper to taste
- 1 (16 ounce) package silken tofu

Directions

- Heat 1 tablespoon of olive oil in a skillet over medium heat. Stir in the garlic and onion; cook and stir until the onion has softened andturned translucent, about 5 minutes. Set aside. Heat the remaining 3tablespoons of olive oil in a large pot over medium-high heat. Stir in the celery, carrots, bell pepper, beets including the greens, whole tomatoes, diced tomatoes, potatoes, Swiss chard, and the onion mixture. Cook and stir until the chard begins to wilt, 4 to 8 minutes. Stir in the vegetable broth, water, dill weed, and salt and pepper.

- Bring to a boil, and reduce heat to low. Simmer for 1 hour.

- Strain half the beets from the broth and place in a blender, filling thepitcher no more than halfway full. Hold down the lid of the blender with a folded kitchen towel, and carefully start the blender, using a few quick pulses to get the beets moving before leaving it on to puree. Add the tofu, and continue pureeing until smooth. Stir the tofu mixture back into the pot. Simmer until the mixture is reduced by a third, about another hour. Serve chilled or warm.

Vegan Yogurt Sundae

Ingredients

- 1/4 cup frozen berries

- tablespoon white sugar
- tablespoons vegan chocolate chips
- 1 tablespoon vegan margarine
- 3 tablespoons soy milk or soy creamer
- 1 (8 ounce) container vanilla soy yogurt
- 1 tablespoon chopped nuts

Directions

- Toss berries with sugar in a microwave safe bowl. Cook in the microwave for 40 seconds at full power until thawed.

- Place chocolate chips and margarine in a microwave safe bowl. Cook in the microwave at 60% power for 45 seconds until melted. Use a fork to stir until smooth, then stir in soy milk until incorporated; set aside.

- Spoon the soy yogurt into a small bowl, then spoon fruit overtop. Pour on chocolate sauce and sprinkle with nuts.

Vegan Pumpkin Ice Cream

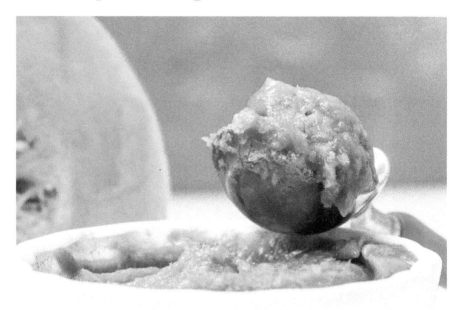

Ingredients

- 1/4 cup soy creamer
- 2 tablespoons arrowroot powder
- 1. 3/4 cups soy creamer
- 1 cup soy milk
- 3/4 cup brown sugar
- 1 cup pumpkin puree
- 1 teaspoon vanilla extract
- 1 1/2 teaspoons pumpkin pie spice

Directions

- Mix 1/4 cup soy creamer with arrowroot and set aside. Whisk together 1 3/4 cup soy creamer, soy milk, brown sugar, pumpkin puree, vanilla extract, and pumpkin pie spice in a saucepan over medium heat, stirring frequently, until just boiling. Remove the pan from the heat; stir in the arrowroot mixture to thicken. Set aside to cool for 30 minutes.

- Fill cylinder of ice cream freezer; freeze according to manufacturer's directions.

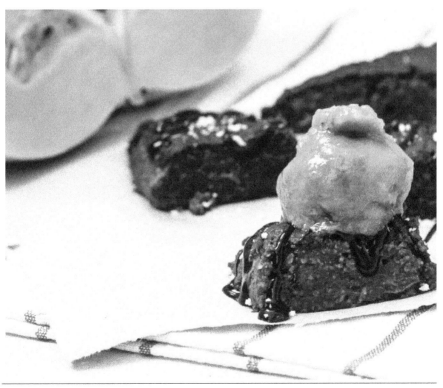

Vegan Chunky Chili

Ingredients

- 1/2 cup dry kidney beans, soaked overnight
- 1/2 cup dry white beans, soaked overnight
- 1/2 cup dry brown lentils, soaked overnight
- 6 cups chopped fresh tomatoes
- 1 cup chopped fresh mushrooms
- 1/2 cup chopped green bell pepper
- 1/2 cup chopped red bell pepper
- 1/2 cup chopped celery
- 1/4 onion, chopped
- 1/4 red onion, chopped
- 3/4 cup extra firm tofu, drained, crumbled
- salt to taste
- black pepper to taste onion powder to taste garlic powder to taste chili powder to taste
- 6 cups water
- 1/2 cup fresh green beans

Directions

- Drain and rinse kidney beans, white beans and lentils. Combine in a large pot and cover with water; boil over medium-high to high heat for 1 hour, or until tender.

- Meanwhile, in a large saucepan over high heat, combine tomatoes and water; bring to a boil. Reduce heat to low and simmer, uncovered, for 1 hour, or until tomatoes are broken down.

- Stir the tomatoes into the beans and add mushrooms, green bell pepper, red bell pepper, green beans, celery, onions and tofu.
- Season with salt, pepper, onion powder, garlic powder and chili powder to taste. Simmer for 2 to 3 hours, or until desired consistency is reached.

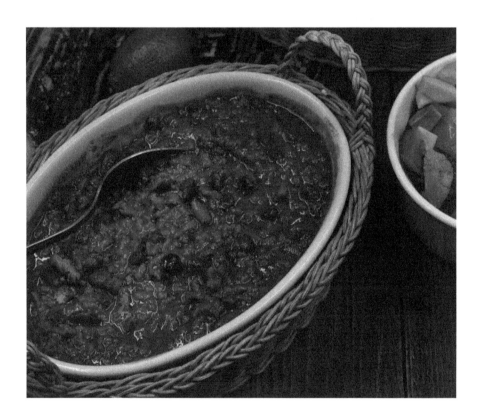

Vegan Lasagna II

Ingredients

- 2/3 (16 ounce) package instant lasagna noodles
- 3 cloves garlic, minced
- 1/2 pound mushrooms
- 1 tablespoon vegetable oil
- (10.75 ounce) can tomato puree

- (10 ounce) package frozen spinach, thawed and drained
- 2 teaspoons garlic salt
- tablespoons Italian-style seasoning
- 1 (12 ounce) package soft tofu

Directions

- Preheat oven to 375 degrees F (190 degrees C).

- In a large skillet, saute garlic and mushrooms in oil until all the liquidis cooked out. Add 1/3 tomato puree to mushrooms and garlic, cook 2 to 3 minutes, and remove from heat.

- In a microwave-safe bowl, combine spinach, garlic salt, Italian seasoning and tofu. Blend until the mixture is an even consistency.Heat in a microwave on high for 2 minutes.

- In a 9x9 inch baking pan, pour one thin layer of remaining tomatopuree, a layer of noodles, 1/2 the tofu mixture, the mushroom sauce, a layer of noodles, 1/2 the tofu mixture, a layer of tomato puree, a layer of noodles, and a final layer of tomato puree.

- Bake 45 minutes in the preheated oven.

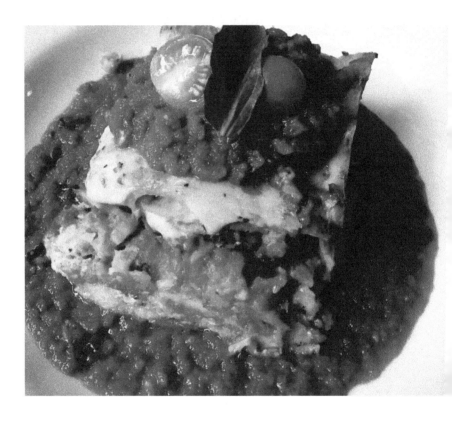

Vegan Carrot Cake

Ingredients

- 2 cups whole wheat flour
- 1/4 cup soy flour (optional)
- 1. 1/2 tablespoons ground cinnamon

- tablespoon ground cloves 4 teaspoons baking soda
- teaspoons tapioca starch (optional)
- 1/2 teaspoon salt

- 1/2 cups hot water
- 1/4 cup flax seed meal
- cups packed brown sugar
- 4 teaspoons vanilla extract
- 3/4 cup dried currants (optional)
- 6 carrots, grated
- 1/2 cup blanched slivered almonds (optional)

Directions

- Preheat oven to 350 degrees F (175 degrees C). Prepare a 9x13inch baking pan with cooking spray. Whisk together the whole wheat flour, soy flour, cinnamon, ground cloves, baking soda, tapioca starch, and salt in a bowl until blended; set aside.

- Pour the hot water into a mixing bowl, and sprinkle with the flax meal. Stir for a minute until the flax begins to absorb the water, and the mixture slightly thickens. Stir in the brown sugar and vanilla until the sugar has dissolved, then add the currants, carrots, and almonds. Stir in the dry mixture until just moistened, then pour into
- the prepared pan

- Bake in the preheated oven until a toothpick inserted into the centercomes out clean, about 30 minutes. Cool in the pan for 10 minutes before removing to cool completely on a wire rack.

Garbage Salad

Ingredients

- 1 head iceberg lettuce
- 1 head romaine lettuce
- 2 tomatoes, cut into chunks
- 1 (14-ounce) can hearts of palm, drained and cut
- 1 (14-ounce) can artichoke hearts, drained and quartered
- 1 (7-ounce) jar roasted red peppers, drained and cut into strips
- 1 (5.75-ounce) can large pitted black olives, drained
- 1 (16-ounce) jar peperoncini, drained
- 2 1/2 cups prepared vinaigrette dressing

Directions

- Wash and dry lettuce and tomatoes then cut into bite-sized pieces. Place in a very large mixing bowl with remaining ingredients except dressing; toss to mix well.

- Pour desired amount of dressing over salad; toss to coat. Serve immediately.

Cinnamon Maple Roasted Veggies

Ingredients

- 1/4 cup vegetable oil
- 1/2 teaspoon ground cinnamon
- 1 teaspoon salt
- 1/4 teaspoon black pepper
- 1 1/2 pounds butternut squash, peeled, seeded, and cut into 1/2-inch cubes
- 1 pound fresh Brussels sprouts, trimmed and cut in half
- 1/2 cup walnut halves
- 1/2 cup dried cranberries
- 3 tablespoons maple syrup

Directions

- Preheat oven to 400 degrees F. In a large bowl, combine oil, cinnamon, salt, and pepper; mix well.

- Add squash and Brussels sprouts and toss until evenly coated. Place vegetable mixture on baking sheets.

- Bake 30 minutes, or until vegetables are tender and begin to brown. Place on a large platter, then sprinkle with walnuts and dried cranberries. Drizzle with syrup and toss gently. Serve immediately.

Vegetarian Bean Chili

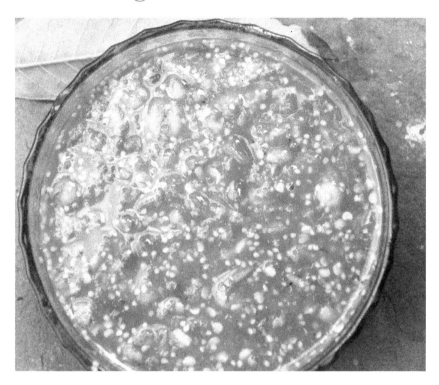

Ingredients

- 2 tablespoons olive oil
- 1 large onion, chopped
- 1 cup picante sauce
- 1 cup vegetable broth
- 2 (28-ounce) cans crushed tomatoes
- 1 (15-ounce) can pinto beans, drained
- 1 (15-ounce) can red kidney beans, drained
- 1 (15-ounce) can black-eyed peas, drained
- 1 teaspoon cumin

Directions

- In a large saucepan or Dutch oven, heat olive oil over medium-high heat; add onion and saute until softened.

- Add remaining ingredients, bring to a boil, then reduce heat and simmer 35 to 40 minutes or until thickened, stirring occasionally.

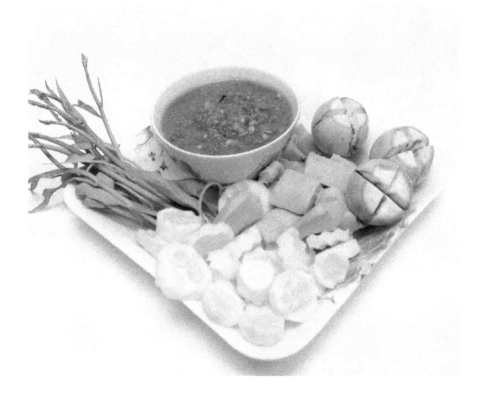

Veggie Chili

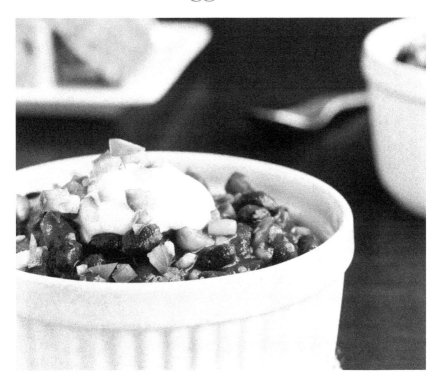

Ingredients

- 1 tablespoon vegetable oil
- 1 large onion, chopped
- 1 (28-ounce) can crushed tomatoes
- 1 cup salsa
- 2 large green bell peppers, cut into 1/2-inch chunks
- 1 1/2 teaspoons chili powder
- 1 1/2 teaspoons ground cumin
- 3/4 teaspoon salt
- 2 (15-ounce) cans black beans, rinsed and drained
- 2 cups frozen corn

Directions

- In a soup pot, heat oil over medium heat. Add onion and sauté 2 to 3 minutes, or until tender. Add tomatoes, salsa, green pepper, chili powder, cumin, and salt; mix well. Reduce heat to low, cover, and simmer 15 minutes.

- Add remaining ingredients, cover, and simmer an additional 15 minutes, or until vegetables are tender. Ladle into bowls and serve.

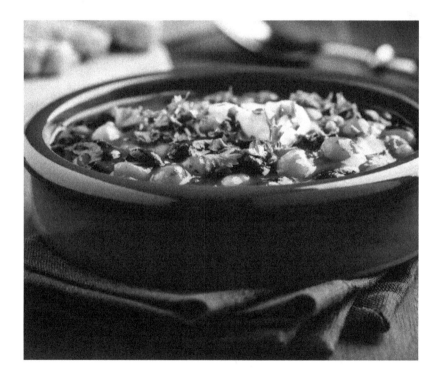

Sweet Potato Black Bean Chili

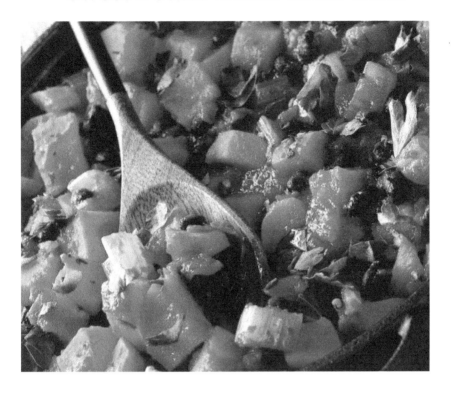

Ingredients

- 3 sweet potatoes, peeled and diced
- 1 red bell pepper, diced
- 1 onion, diced
- 2 (14-1/2-ounce) cans diced tomatoes, undrained
- 2 (15-1/4-ounce) cans black beans, undrained
- 1 tablespoon chili powder
- 2 teaspoons cumin
- 1 teaspoon salt
- 1/2 teaspoon black pepper

Directions

- In a large slow cooker, combine all ingredients; mix well.

- Cover and cook on high 4 hours, or until potatoes are fork-tender.

Veggie Packed Chili

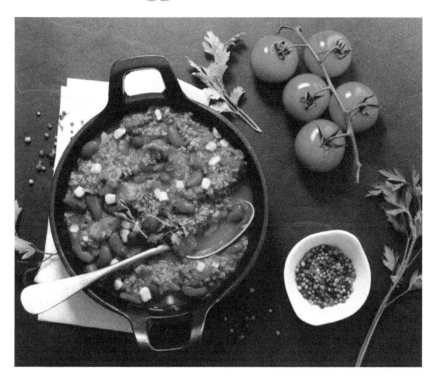

Ingredients

- 1 tablespoon vegetable oil
- 1 large onion, chopped
- 1 (28-ounce) can crushed tomatoes
- 1 cup water
- 2/3 cup salsa (see Note)
- 1 1/2 teaspoons chili powder
- 1 1/2 teaspoons ground cumin
- 3/4 teaspoon salt
- 2 (15-ounce) cans black beans, rinsed and drained
- 1 large green bell pepper, cut into 1/2-inch chunks
- 1 large zucchini, cut into 1/2-inch chunks
- 8 ounces sliced mushrooms

Directions

- In a soup pot, heat oil over medium heat. Add onion and sauté 4 to 5 minutes, or until tender.

- Add remaining ingredients and bring to a boil. Reduce heat to low and simmer for 40 to 45 minutes, or until vegetables are tender. Ladle into bowls and serve.

CPSIA information can be obtained
at www.ICGtesting.com
Printed in the USA
BVHW061253020621
608627BV00008B/552